DASH DIET COO
2021

HOW TO LOWER YOUR BLOOD PRESSURE WITH LOW SODIUM RECIPES AND A 30-DAY MEAL PLAN

Table of Contents

Introduction

Dietary Approaches to Stop Hypertension is one of the most effective organic treatments of all health problems related to high blood pressure or fluid build-up in the body. These approaches come with a complete program, which places emphasis on the diet as well as lifestyle changes. Commonly called the DASH diet, which is the acronym for Dietary Approaches to Stop Hypertension, the major target is to reduce the sodium content of your diet by omitting table salt directly or reducing the intake through other ingredients. There are two minerals that work against each other to maintain the body fluid balance; those are sodium and potassium. In perfect proportions, these two control the release and retention of fluids in the body. In the case of environmental or genetic complexities or a high sodium diet, the balance is disturbed so much that it puts our heart at risk by elevating systolic and diastolic blood pressures.

Origin of the DASH Diet

This dietary plan came to the knowledge of nutritionists after several research studies were conducted to treat hypertension focused on diet in order to avoid medication's side effects. It was seen as a way to reduce blood pressure by using healthy, nourishing food and following an active routine. The main goal was to cure hypertension, so it was soon termed the Dietary Approaches to Stop Hypertension (DASH). However, its broad-scale effects showed greater efficiency than just reducing hypertension, and people started using it to treat obesity, diabetes, cancer, and cardiac disorders.

To study the impact of sodium intake, a scientist used three experimental groups. Each group was assigned a diet with varying sodium levels. One was to take 3300 mg sodium per day; the second had to use 2300 mg per day, and the third one was put on a diet having 1500 mg sodium per day, about two-thirds of a teaspoon of salt. By restricting the sodium content, all participants showed decreased blood pressure. But the group with the least amount of sodium intake showed the most alleviation in the blood pressure levels. Thus, it was identified that 1500 mg of sodium per day is the threshold amount to maintain blood pressure.

The Benefits of the DASH Diet

Besides hypertension, there are several health advantages that later came to light as experts recorded the conditions people experience after choosing the diet. Here are some of the known benefits of the DASH diet:

1. Alleviated Blood Pressure

It is the most obvious and direct outcome of this dietary routine as it restricts sodium intake, which rightly reduces the risks of high blood pressure by keeping the blood consistency near normal. People with hypertension disorder should restrict sodium intake the most, whereas others should keep the intake as per the described limits, 1500 mg per day.

2. Maintained Cholesterol Levels

Since a DASH diet promotes greater use of vegetables, fruits, whole grains, beans, and nuts, it can provide enough fibers to regulate our metabolism and digestive functions. Moreover, it promotes only lean meats and no saturated fats, which also helps maintain cholesterol levels in the body. Such fats have to be replaced with healthy cholesterol fats to keep the heart running.

3. Weight Maintenance

Weight loss is another primary objective for people on the DASH diet. With a nutritious and clean diet, anyone can lose excess weight. Moreover, the DASH diet also promotes proper physical exercise every day, which also proves to be significant in reducing obesity. Sometimes, obesity is the result of inflammation or fluid imbalances in the body, and the DASH diet can even cure that through its progressive health approach.

4. Reduced Risks of Osteoporosis

Osteoporosis is the degeneration of the bones, and there are many factors associated with it; at the base of it is the decrease of calcium and vitamin D in the body. The DASH diet provides ways and meals to fill this deficiency gap and reduce the risks of osteoporosis, especially in women.

5. Healthier Kidneys

Kidneys are what control the fluid balance of the body with the help of hormones and minerals. So, a smart diet designed with the sole purpose of aiding kidney functions can keep them healthy and functioning properly. Excess salt or oxalate intake can cause kidney stones. The DASH diet reduces the chances of these stones from building up in the kidneys.

6. Protection from Cancers

The DASH diet has been proven effective in preventing people from different types of cancers, like kidney, lung, prostate, esophagus, rectum, and colon cancers. The diet co-joins all the important factors which can fight against cancer and help prevent the development of cancerous cells.

7. Prevention of Diabetes

The DASH diet is effective in reducing insulin resistance, which is one of the common causes of diabetes in many people. Reduced weight, an active metabolism, maintained body fluids, daily exercises, increased water consumption, a low sodium diet, and a healthy gut or digestive system are all the factors that link the DASH diet with the reduced risks of diabetes in a person.

8. Improved Mental Health

Mental health is largely dependent on the type of food you eat. Anxiety, depression, and insomnia are all outcomes of poor health and a bad lifestyle. The entire neural transmission is controlled by the electrolyte balance in the nervous system. With the DASH diet, you can create optimum conditions for efficient brain functions.

9. Less Risk of Heart Disease

Since the DASH diet is designed to control varying blood pressure, it saves the heart from the negative impact of high blood pressure and prevents it from different diseases. Constant high blood pressure burdens the heart and causes the weakening of its walls and valves. Such risks are reduced with the help of the DASH diet.

30 Day Meal Plan

Day	Breakfast	Lunch	Dinner	Dessert
1	Greek Yogurt Oat Pancakes	Creamy Pumpkin Pasta	Oregano Chicken Thighs	Banana-Cashew Cream Mousse
2	Chia Seeds Breakfast Mix	Steamed Fish Mediterranean Style	Spicy Tofu Burrito Bowls with Cilantro Avocado Sauce	Grilled Pineapple Strips
3	Creamy Oats, Greens & Blueberry Smoothie	Steamed Tilapia with Green Chutney	Harissa Bolognese with Vegetable Noodles	Mango Rice Pudding
4	Turkey Sausage and Mushroom Strata	Pumpkin and Black Beans Chicken	Eggplant Parmesan Stacks	Grilled Plums with Vanilla Bean Frozen Yogurt
5	Scrambled Egg and Veggie Breakfast Quesadillas	Mexican-Style Potato Casserole	Teriyaki Chicken Wings	Apple Dumplings
6	Peanut Butter & Banana Breakfast Smoothie	Rosemary Roasted Chicken	Poached Salmon with Creamy Piccata Sauce	Homemade Banana Ice Cream
7	Spinach, Mushroom, and Feta Cheese Scramble	White Beans with Spinach and Pan-Roasted Tomatoes	Pesto Chicken Breasts with Summer Squash	Key Lime Cherry "Nice" Cream

8	Banana & Cinnamon Oatmeal	Healthy Chicken Orzo	Quick Shrimp Scampi	Choco Banana Cake
9	Sweet Potato Toast Three Ways	Grilled Mahi-Mahi with Artichoke Caponata	Hot Chicken Wings	Carrot Cake Cookies
10	Steel Cut Oat Blueberry Pancakes	Mediterranean Turkey Breast	Tuna Salad-Stuffed Tomatoes with Arugula	Ginger Snaps
11	Turkey Sausage and Mushroom Strata	Steamed Fish Mediterranean Style	Harissa Bolognese with Vegetable Noodles	Grilled Plums with Vanilla Bean Frozen Yogurt
12	Peanut Butter & Banana Breakfast Smoothie	Steamed Tilapia with Green Chutney	Oregano Chicken Thighs	Banana-Cashew Cream Mousse
13	Chia Seeds Breakfast Mix	Rosemary Roasted Chicken	Poached Salmon with Creamy Piccata Sauce	Key Lime Cherry "Nice" Cream
14	Banana & Cinnamon Oatmeal	Grilled Mahi-Mahi with Artichoke Caponata	Teriyaki Chicken Wings	Apple Dumplings
15	Scrambled Egg and Veggie Breakfast Quesadillas	Pumpkin and Black Beans Chicken	Eggplant Parmesan Stacks	Carrot Cake Cookies

16	Steel Cut Oat Blueberry Pancakes	Mediterranean Turkey Breast	Spicy Tofu Burrito Bowls with Cilantro Avocado Sauce	Homemade Banana Ice Cream
17	Creamy Oats, Greens & Blueberry Smoothie	Mexican-Style Potato Casserole	Hot Chicken Wings	Choco Banana Cake
18	Sweet Potato Toast Three Ways	Healthy Chicken Orzo	Tuna Salad-Stuffed Tomatoes with Arugula	Mango Rice Pudding
19	Spinach, Mushroom, and Feta Cheese Scramble	White Beans with Spinach and Pan-Roasted Tomatoes	Quick Shrimp Scampi	Ginger Snaps
20	Greek Yogurt Oat Pancakes	Creamy Pumpkin Pasta	Pesto Chicken Breasts with Summer Squash	Grilled Pineapple Strips
21	Chia Seeds Breakfast Mix	Steamed Fish Mediterranean Style	Oregano Chicken Thighs	Apple Dumplings
22	Peanut Butter & Banana Breakfast Smoothie	Rosemary Roasted Chicken	Poached Salmon with Creamy Piccata Sauce	Banana-Cashew Cream Mousse
23	Turkey Sausage and Mushroom Strata	Pumpkin and Black Beans Chicken	Harissa Bolognese with Vegetable Noodles	Grilled Plums with Vanilla Bean Frozen Yogurt

24	Banana & Cinnamon Oatmeal	Steamed Tilapia with Green Chutney	Eggplant Parmesan Stacks	Choco Banana Cake
25	Creamy Oats, Greens & Blueberry Smoothie	Mediterranean Turkey Breast	Tuna Salad-Stuffed Tomatoes with Arugula	Grilled Pineapple Strips
26	Scrambled Egg and Veggie Breakfast Quesadillas	Mexican-Style Potato Casserole	Teriyaki Chicken Wings	Ginger Snaps
27	Steel Cut Oat Blueberry Pancakes	Creamy Pumpkin Pasta	Spicy Tofu Burrito Bowls with Cilantro Avocado Sauce	Mango Rice Pudding
28	Greek Yogurt Oat Pancakes	Grilled Mahi-Mahi with Artichoke Caponata	Hot Chicken Wings	Key Lime Cherry "Nice" Cream
29	Sweet Potato Toast Three Ways	Healthy Chicken Orzo	Quick Shrimp Scampi	Carrot Cake Cookies
30	Spinach, Mushroom, and Feta Cheese Scramble	White Beans with Spinach and Pan-Roasted Tomatoes	Pesto Chicken Breasts with Summer Squash	Homemade Banana Ice Cream

1. Oatmeal Banana Pancakes with Walnuts

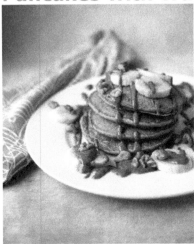

Preparation Time: 15 minutes
Cooking Time: 5 minutes
Servings: 8
Ingredients:

- 1 finely diced firm banana
- 1 c. whole wheat pancake mix
- 1/8 c. chopped walnuts
- ¼ c. old-fashioned oats

Directions:

1. Make the pancake mix, as stated in the directions on the package. Add walnuts, oats, and chopped banana. Coat a griddle with cooking spray. Add about ¼ cup of the pancake batter onto the griddle when hot.
2. Turn pancake over when bubbles form on top. Cook until golden brown. Serve immediately.

Nutrition:

- Calories: 155
- Fat: 4 g
- Carbs: 28 g
- Protein: 7 g
- Sugars: 2.2 g
- Sodium: 16 mg

2. Creamy Oats, Greens & Blueberry Smoothie

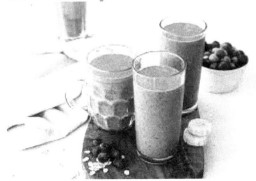

Preparation Time: 4 minutes
Cooking Time: 0 minutes
Servings: 1
Ingredients:

- 1 c. cold
- Fat-free milk
- 1 c. salad greens
- ½ c. fresh frozen blueberries
- ½ c. frozen cooked oatmeal
- 1 tbsp. sunflower seeds

Directions:

1. Blend all ingredients using a powerful blender until smooth and creamy. Serve and enjoy.

Nutrition:

- Calories: 280
- Fat: 6.8 g
- Carbs: 44.0 g
- Protein: 14.0 g
- Sugars: 32 g
- Sodium: 141 mg

3. Greek Yogurt Oat Pancakes

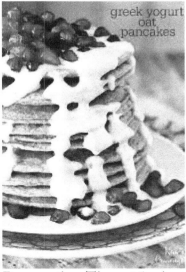

Preparation Time: 15 minutes
Cooking Time: 10 minutes
Servings: 2
Ingredients:

- 6 egg whites (or ¾ cup liquid egg whites)
- 1 cup rolled oats
- 1 cup plain nonfat Greek yogurt
- 1 medium banana, peeled and sliced
- 1 teaspoon ground cinnamon
- 1 teaspoon baking powder

Directions:
1. Blend all of the listed ingredients using a blender. Warm a griddle over medium heat. Spray the skillet with nonstick cooking spray.
2. Put 1/3 cup of the mixture or batter onto the griddle. Allow to cook and flip when bubbles on the top burst, about 5 minutes. Cook again for a minute until golden brown. Repeat with the remaining batter. Divide between two serving plates and enjoy.

Nutrition:
- Calories: 318
- Fat: 4g
- Sodium: 467mg
- Potassium: 634mg
- Carbohydrates: 47g
- Fiber: 6g
- Sugars: 13g
- Protein: 28g

4. Scrambled Egg and Veggie Breakfast Quesadillas

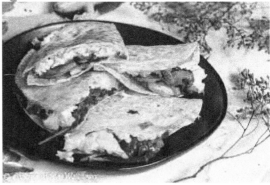

Preparation Time: 15 minutes
Cooking Time: 15 minutes
Servings: 2
Ingredients:

- 2 egg1s
- 2 egg whites
- 2 to 4 tablespoons nonfat or low-fat milk
- ¼ teaspoon freshly ground black pepper
- 1 large tomato, chopped
- 2 tablespoons chopped cilantro
- ½ cup canned black beans, rinsed and drained
- 1½ tablespoons olive oil, divided
- 4 corn tortillas
- ½ avocado, peeled, pitted, and thinly sliced

Directions:
1. Mix the eggs, egg whites, milk, and black pepper in a bowl. Using an electric mixer, beat until smooth. To the same bowl, add the tomato,

cilantro, and black beans, and fold into the eggs with a spoon.

2. Heat half of the olive oil in a medium pan over medium heat. Add the scrambled egg mixture and cook for a few minutes, stirring, until cooked through. Remove from the pan.

3. Divide the scrambled egg mixture between the tortillas, layering only on one half of the tortilla. Top with avocado slices and fold the tortillas in half.

4. Heat the remaining oil over medium heat, and add one of the folded tortillas to the pan. Cook from 1 to 2 minutes on each side or until browned. Repeat with remaining tortillas. Serve immediately.

Nutrition:
- Calories: 445
- Fat: 24g
- Sodium: 228mg
- Potassium: 614mg
- Carbohydrates: 42g
- Fiber: 11g
- Sugars: 2g
- Protein: 19g

5. Stuffed Breakfast Peppers

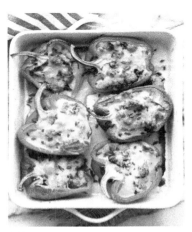

Preparation Time: 15 minutes
Cooking Time: 45 minutes
Servings: 4
Ingredients:
- 4 bell peppers (any color)
- 1 (16-ounce) bag frozen spinach
- 4 eggs
- ¼ cup shredded low-fat cheese (optional)
- Freshly ground black pepper

Directions:

1. Preheat the oven to 400°F. Line a baking dish with aluminum foil. Cut the tops off the pepper, then discard the seeds. Discard the tops and seeds. Put the peppers in the baking dish, and bake for about 15 minutes.

2. While the peppers bake, defrost the spinach and drain off the excess moisture. Remove the peppers, then stuff the bottoms evenly with the defrosted spinach.

3. Crack an egg over the spinach inside each pepper. Top each egg with a tablespoon of the cheese (if using) and season with black pepper to taste. Bake between 15 to 20 minutes, or until the egg whites are set and opaque.

Nutrition:
- Calories: 136
- Fat: 5g
- Sodium: 131mg
- Potassium: 576mg
- Carbohydrates: 15g
- Protein: 11g

6. Sweet Potato Toast Three Ways

SWEET POTATO TOAST

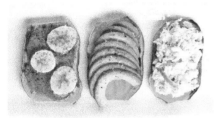

3 Ways!

Preparation Time: 15 minutes
Cooking Time: 2 5 minutes
Servings:
Ingredients:
- 1 large sweet potato, unpeeled

Topping Choice #1:
- 4 tablespoons peanut butter
- 1 ripe banana, sliced
- Dash ground cinnamon

Topping Choice #2:
- ½ avocado, peeled, pitted, and mashed
- 2 eggs (1 per slice)
- Topping Choice #3:
- 4 tablespoons nonfat or low-fat ricotta cheese
- 1 tomato, sliced
- Dash black pepper

Directions:
1. Slice the sweet potato lengthwise into ¼-inch thick slices. Place the sweet potato slices in a toaster on high for about 5 minutes or until cooked through.
2. Repeat multiple times, if necessary, depending on your toaster settings. Top with your desired topping choices and enjoy.
Nutrition:

- Calories: 137
- Fat: 0g
- Sodium: 17mg
- Potassium: 265mg
- Carbohydrates: 32g
- Fiber: 4g
- Sugars: 0g
- Protein: 2g

7. Pineapple Oatmeal

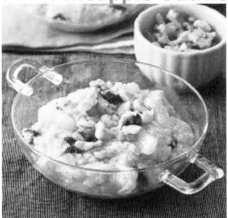

Preparation Time: 10 minutes
Cooking Time: 25 minutes
Servings: 4
Ingredients:
- 2 cups old-fashioned oats
- 1 cup walnuts, chopped
- 2 cups pineapple, cubed
- 1 tablespoon ginger, grated
- 2 cups non-fat milk
- 2 eggs
- 2 tablespoons stevia
- 2 teaspoons vanilla extract

Directions:
1. In a bowl, combine the oats with the pineapple, walnuts, and ginger, stir and divide into 4 ramekins. Mix the milk with the eggs, stevia, and vanilla in a bowl and pour over the oats mix. Bake at 400 degrees F for 25 minutes. Serve for breakfast.

Nutrition:
- Calories: 200
- Carbs: 40g
- Fat: 1g
- Protein: 3g
- Sodium: 275 mg

8. Spinach Muffins

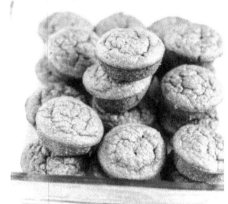

Preparation Time: 10 minutes
Cooking Time: 30 minutes
Servings: 6
Ingredients:
- 6 eggs
- ½ cup non-fat milk
- 1 cup low-fat cheese, crumbled
- 4 ounces spinach
- ½ cup roasted red pepper, chopped
- 2 ounces prosciutto, chopped
- Cooking spray

Directions:
1. Mix the eggs with the milk, cheese, spinach, red pepper, and prosciutto in a bowl. Grease a muffin tray with cooking spray, divide the muffin mix, introduce in the oven, and bake at 350 degrees F for 30 minutes. Divide between plates and serve for breakfast.

Nutrition:
- Calories: 112

- Carbs: 19g
- Fat: 3g
- Protein: 2g
- Sodium: 274 mg

9. Chia Seeds Breakfast Mix

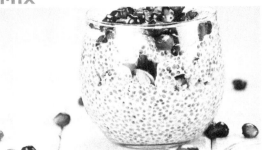

Preparation Time: 8 hours
Cooking Time: 0 minutes
Servings: 4
Ingredients:
- 2 cups old-fashioned oats
- 4 tablespoons chia seeds
- 4 tablespoons coconut sugar
- 3 cups of coconut milk
- 1 teaspoon lemon zest, grated
- 1 cup blueberries

Directions:
1. In a bowl, combine the oats with chia seeds, sugar, milk, lemon zest, and blueberries, stir, divide into cups and keep in the fridge for 8 hours.
2. Serve for breakfast.

Nutrition:
- Calories: 69
- Carbs: 0g
- Fat: 5g
- Protein: 3g
- Sodium: 0 mg

10. Breakfast Fruits Bowls

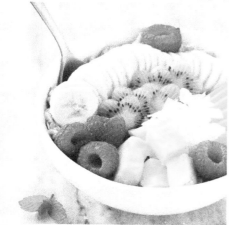

Preparation Time: 10 minutes
Cooking Time: 0 minutes
Servings: 2
Ingredients:

- 1 cup mango, chopped
- 1 banana, sliced
- 1 cup pineapple, chopped
- 1 cup almond milk

Directions:
1.   Mix the mango with the banana, pineapple, and almond milk in a bowl, stir, divide into smaller bowls, and serve.

Nutrition:

- Calories: 10
- Carbs: 0g
- Fat: 1g
- Protein: 0g
- Sodium: 0mg

11. Pesto Omelet

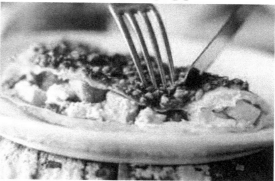

Preparation Time: 10 minutes
Cooking Time: 6 minutes
Servings: 2
Ingredients:

- 2 teaspoons olive oil
- Handful cherry tomatoes, chopped
- 3 tablespoons pistachio pesto
- A pinch of black pepper
- 4 eggs

Directions:
1.   In a bowl, combine the eggs with cherry tomatoes, black pepper, and pistachio pesto and whisk well. Add egg mix, spread into the pan, cook for 3 minutes, flip, cook for 3 minutes more, divide between 2 plates, and serve on a heated pan with the oil over medium-high heat.

Nutrition:

- Calories: 240
- Carbs: 23g
- Fat: 9g
- Protein: 17g
- Sodium: 292 mg

12. Quinoa Bowls

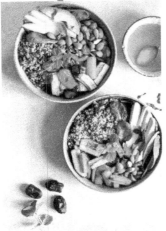

Preparation Time: 10 minutes
Cooking Time: 20 minutes
Servings: 2
Ingredients:

- 1 peach, sliced
- 1/3 cup quinoa, rinsed
- 2/3 cup low-fat milk
- ½ teaspoon vanilla extract
- 2 teaspoons brown sugar
- 12 raspberries
- 14 blueberries

Directions:

1. Mix the quinoa with the milk, sugar, and vanilla in a small pan, simmer over medium heat, cover the pan, cook for 20 minutes and flip with a fork. Divide this mix into 2 bowls, top each with raspberries and blueberries, and serve for breakfast.

Nutrition:

- Calories: 170
- Carbs: 31g
- Fat: 3g
- Protein: 6g
- Sodium: 120 mg

13. Strawberry Sandwich

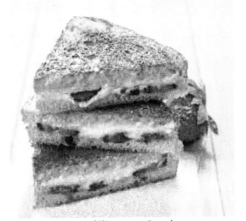

Preparation Time: 10 minutes
Cooking Time: 0 minutes
Servings: 4
Ingredients:

- 8 ounces low-fat cream cheese, soft
- 1 tablespoon stevia
- 1 teaspoon lemon zest, grated
- 4 whole-wheat English muffins, toasted
- 2 cups strawberries, sliced

Directions:

1. In your food processor, combine the cream cheese with the stevia and lemon zest and pulse well. Spread 1 tablespoon of this mix on 1 muffin half and top with some of the sliced strawberries. Repeat with the rest of the muffin halves and serve for breakfast. Enjoy!

Nutrition:

- Calories: 150
- Carbs: 23g
- Fat: 7g
- Protein: 2g
- Sodium: 70 mg

14. Turkey Sausage and Mushroom Strata

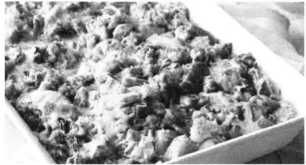

Preparation Time: 15 minutes
Cooking Time: 8 minutes
Servings: 12
Ingredients:

- 8 oz. cubed Ciabatta bread
- 12 oz. chopped turkey sausage
- 2 c. Milk
- 4 oz. shredded Cheddar
- 3 large Eggs
- 12 oz. Egg substitute
- ½ c. chopped Green onion
- 1 c. diced Mushroom
- ½ tsp. Paprika
- ½ tsp. Pepper
- 2 tbsps. grated Parmesan cheese

Directions:

1. Set oven to preheat to 400F. Lay your bread cubes flat on a baking tray and set it to toast for about 8 min. Meanwhile, add a skillet over medium heat with sausage and cook while stirring until fully brown and crumbled.
2. Mix salt, pepper, paprika, parmesan cheese, egg substitute, eggs, cheddar cheese, and milk in a large bowl. Add in your remaining ingredients and toss well to incorporate.
3. Transfer mixture to a large baking dish (preferably a 9x13-inch), then tightly cover and allow to rest in the refrigerator overnight. Set your oven to preheat to 350F, remove the cover from your casserole, and set to bake until golden brown and cooked through. Slice and serve.

Nutrition:

- Calories: 288.2
- Protein 24.3g
- Carbs 18.2g
- Fat. 12.4g
- Sodium 355 mg

15. Bacon Bits

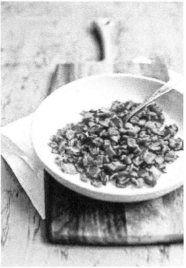

Preparation Time: 15 minutes
Cooking Time: 60 minutes
Servings: 4
Ingredients:

- 1 c. Millet
- 5 c. Water
- 1 c. diced Sweet potato
- 1 tsp. ground Cinnamon
- 2 tbsps. Brown sugar
- 1 medium diced Apple
- ¼ c. Honey

Directions:

1. In a deep pot, add your sugar, sweet potato, cinnamon, water, and millet, then stir to combine, then boil on high heat. After that, simmer on low.

2. Cook like this for about an hour until your water is fully absorbed and millet is cooked. Stir in your remaining ingredients and serve.

Nutrition:
- Calories: 136
- Protein 3.1g
- Carbs 28.5g
- Fat 1.0g
- Sodium 120 mg

16. Steel Cut Oat Blueberry Pancakes

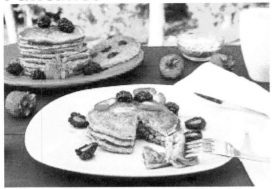

Preparation Time: 15 minutes
Cooking Time: 15 minutes
Servings: 4
Ingredients:
- 1½ c. Water
- ½ c. steel-cut oats
- 1/8 tsp. Salt
- 1 c. Whole wheat Flour
- ½ tsp. Baking powder
- ½ tsp. Baking soda
- 1 Egg
- 1 c. Milk
- ½ c. Greek yogurt
- 1 c. Frozen Blueberries
- ¾ c. Agave Nectar

Directions:
1. Combine your oats, salt, and water in a medium saucepan, stir, and allow to come to a boil over high heat. Adjust the heat to low, and allow to simmer for about 10 min, or until oats get tender. Set aside.
2. Combine all your remaining ingredients, except agave nectar, in a medium bowl, then fold in oats. Preheat your skillet and lightly grease it. Cook ¼ cup of milk batter at a time for about 3 minutes per side. Garnish with Agave Nectar.

Nutrition:
- Calories: 257
- Protein 14g
- Carbs 46g
- Fat 7g
- Sodium 123 mg

17. Spinach, Mushroom, and Feta Cheese Scramble

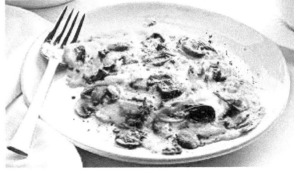

Preparation Time: 15 minutes
Cooking Time: 4 minutes
Servings: 1
Ingredients:
- Olive oil cooking spray
- ½ c. sliced Mushroom
- 1 c. chopped Spinach
- 3 Eggs
- 2 tbsps. Feta cheese
- Pepper

Directions:

1. Set a lightly greased medium skillet over medium heat. Add spinach and mushrooms, and cook until spinach wilts.

2. Combine egg whites, cheese, pepper, and whole egg in a medium bowl, whisk to combine. Pour into your skillet and cook, while stirring, until set (about 4 minutes). Serve.

Nutrition:

- Calories: 236.5
- Protein 22.2g
- Carbs 12.9g
- Fat 11.4g
- Sodium 405 mg

18. Red Velvet Pancakes with Cream Cheese Topping

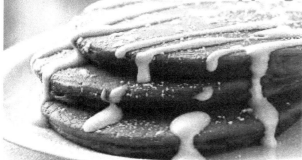

Preparation Time: 15 minutes
Cooking Time: 10 minutes
Servings: 2
Ingredients:
Cream Cheese Topping:

- 2 oz. Cream cheese
- 3 tbsps. Yogurt
- 3 tbsps. Honey
- 1 tbsp. Milk

Pancakes:

- ½ c. Whole wheat Flour
- ½ c. all-purpose flour
- 2¼tsps. Baking powder
- ½ tsp. Unsweetened Cocoa powder
- ¼ tsp. Salt
- ¼ c. Sugar

- 1 large Egg
- 1 c. + 2 tbsps. Milk
- 1 tsp. Vanilla
- 1 tsp. Red paste food coloring

Directions:

1. Combine all your topping ingredients in a medium bowl, and set aside. Add all your pancake ingredients to a large bowl and fold until combined. Set a greased skillet over medium heat to get hot.

2. Add ¼ cup of pancake batter onto the hot skillet and cook until bubbles begin to form on the top. Flip and cook until set. Repeat until your batter is done well. Add your toppings and serve.

Nutrition:

- Calories: 231
- Protein 7g
- Carbs 43g
- Fat 4g
- Sodium 0mg

19. Peanut Butter & Banana Breakfast Smoothie

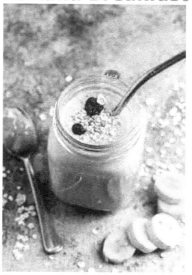

Preparation Time: 15 minutes
Cooking Time: 0 minutes

Servings: 1

Ingredients:

- 1 c. Non-fat milk
- 1 tbsp. Peanut butter
- 1 Banana
- ½ tsp. Vanilla

Directions:

1. Place non-fat milk, peanut butter, and banana in a blender. Blend until smooth.

Nutrition:

- Calories: 295
- Protein 133g
- Carbs 42g
- Fat 8.4g
- Sodium 100 mg

20. No-Bake Breakfast Granola Bars

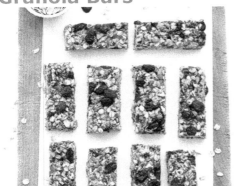

Preparation Time: 15 minutes

Cooking Time: 0 minutes

Servings: 18

Ingredients:

- 2 c. Old fashioned oatmeal
- ½ c. Raisins
- ½ c. Brown sugar
- 2½ c. Corn rice cereal
- ½ c. Syrup
- ½ c. Peanut butter
- ½ tsp. Vanilla

Directions:

1. In a suitable size mixing bowl, mix using a wooden spoon, rice cereal, oatmeal, and raisins. In a saucepan, combine corn syrup and brown sugar. On a medium-high flame, continuously stir the mixture and bring to a boil.

2. On boiling, take away from heat. In a saucepan, stir vanilla and peanut into the sugar mixture. Stir until very smooth.

3. Spoon peanut butter mixture on the cereal and raisins into the mixing bowl and combine — shape mixture into a 9 x 13 baking tin. Allow to cool properly, then cut into bars (18 pcs).

Nutrition:

- Calories: 152
- Protein 4g
- Carbs 26g
- Fat 4.3g
- Sodium 160 mg

21. Pumpkin Cookies

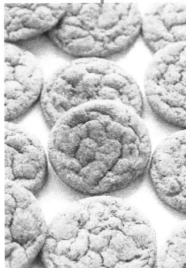

Preparation Time: 10 minutes

Cooking Time: 25 minutes

Servings: 6

Ingredients:

- 2 cups whole wheat flour
- 1 cup old-fashioned oats

- 1 teaspoon baking soda
- 1 teaspoon pumpkin pie spice
- 15 ounces pumpkin puree
- 1 cup coconut oil, melted
- 1 cup of coconut sugar
- 1 egg
- ½ cup pepitas, roasted
- ½ cup cherries, dried

Directions:

1.   Mix the flour the oats, baking soda, pumpkin spice, pumpkin puree, oil, sugar, egg, pepitas, and cherries in a bowl, stir well, shape medium cookies out of this mix, arrange them all on a baking sheet, then bake for 25 minutes at 350 degrees F. Serve the cookies for breakfast.

Nutrition:

- Calories: 150
- Carbs: 24g
- Fat: 8g
- Protein: 1g
- Sodium: 220 mg

22.   Banana & Cinnamon Oatmeal

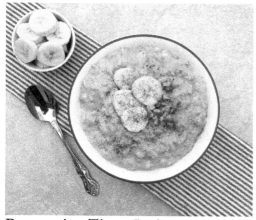

Preparation Time: 5 minutes
Cooking Time: 0 minutes
Servings: 6
Ingredients:

- 2 c. quick-cooking oats
- 4 c. Fat-free milk
- 1 tsp. ground cinnamon
- 2 chopped large ripe banana
- 4 tsp. Brown sugar
- Extra ground cinnamon

Directions:

1.   Place milk in a skillet and bring to boil. Add oats and cook over medium heat until thickened, for two to four minutes.

2.   Stir intermittently. Add cinnamon, brown sugar, and banana and stir to combine. If you want, serve with the extra cinnamon and milk. Enjoy!

Nutrition:

- Calories: 215
- Fat: 2 g
- Carbs: 42 g
- Protein: 10 g
- Sugars: 1 g
- Sodium: 40 mg

23.   Apple Pancakes

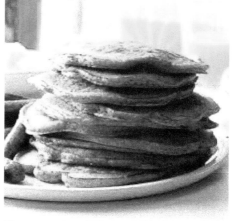

Preparation Time: 15 minutes
Cooking Time: 5 minutes
Servings: 16
Ingredients:

- ¼ cup extra-virgin olive oil, divided
- 1 cup whole wheat flour

- 2 teaspoons baking powder
- 1 teaspoon baking soda
- 1 teaspoon ground cinnamon
- 1 cup 1% milk
- 2 large eggs
- 1 medium Gala apple, diced
- 2 tablespoons maple syrup
- ¼ cup chopped walnuts

Directions:
1.   Set aside 1 teaspoon of oil to use for greasing a griddle or skillet. In a large bowl, stir the flour, baking powder, baking soda, cinnamon, milk, eggs, apple, and the remaining oil.
2.   Warm griddle or skillet on medium-high heat and coat with the reserved oil. Working in batches, pour in about ¼ cup of the batter for each pancake. Cook until browned on both sides.
3.   Place 4 pancakes into each of 4 medium storage containers and the maple syrup in 4 small containers. Put each serving with 1 tablespoon of walnuts and drizzle with ½ tablespoon of maple syrup.

Nutrition:
- Calories: 378
- Fat: 22g
- Carbohydrates: 39g
- Protein: 10g
- Sodium: 65mg

24. Super-Simple Granola

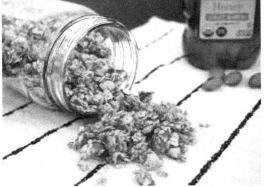

Preparation Time: 15 minutes
Cooking Time: 25 minutes
Servings: 8
Ingredients:
- ¼ cup extra-virgin olive oil
- ¼ cup honey
- ½ teaspoon ground cinnamon
- ½ teaspoon vanilla extract
- ¼ teaspoon salt
- 2 cups rolled oats
- ½ cup chopped walnuts
- ½ cup slivered almonds

Directions:
1.   Preheat the oven to 350°F. Mix the oil, honey, cinnamon, vanilla, and salt in a large bowl. Add the oats, walnuts, and almonds. Stir to coat. Put the batter out onto the prepared sheet pan. Bake for 20 minutes. Let cool.

Nutrition:
- Calories: 254
- Fat: 16g
- Carbohydrates: 25g
- Fiber: 3.5g
- Protein: 5g
- Potassium: 163mg
- Sodium: 73mg

25. Savory Yogurt Bowls

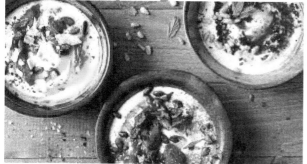

Preparation Time: 15 minutes
Cooking Time: 0 minutes
Servings: 4
Ingredients:

- 1 medium cucumber, diced
- ½ cup pitted Kalamata olives, halved
- 2 tablespoons fresh lemon juice
- 1 tablespoon extra-virgin olive oil
- 1 teaspoon dried oregano
- ¼ teaspoon freshly ground black pepper
- 2 cups nonfat plain Greek yogurt
- ½ cup slivered almonds

Directions:

1.   In a small bowl, mix the cucumber, olives, lemon juice, oil, oregano, and pepper. Divide the yogurt evenly among 4 storage containers. Top with the cucumber-olive mix and almonds.

Nutrition:

- Calories: 240
- Fat: 16g
- Carbohydrates: 10g
- Protein: 16g
- Potassium: 353mg
- Sodium: 350mg

26. Energy Sunrise Muffins

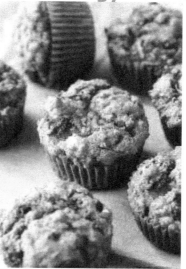

Preparation Time: 15 minutes
Cooking Time: 25 minutes
Servings: 16
Ingredients:

- Nonstick cooking spray
- 2 cups whole wheat flour
- 2 teaspoons baking soda
- 2 teaspoons ground cinnamon
- 1 teaspoon ground ginger
- ¼ teaspoon salt
- 3 large eggs
- ½ cup packed brown sugar
- 1/3 cup unsweetened applesauce
- ¼ cup honey
- ¼ cup vegetable or canola oil
- 1 teaspoon grated orange zest
- Juice of 1 medium orange
- 2 teaspoons vanilla extract
- 2 cups shredded carrots
- 1 large apple, peeled and grated
- ½ cup golden raisins
- ½ cup chopped pecans
- ½ cup unsweetened coconut flakes

Directions:

1. If you can fit two 12-cup muffin tins side by side in your oven, then leave a rack in the middle, then preheat the oven to 350°F.

2. Coat 16 cups of the muffin tins with cooking spray or line with paper liners. Mix the flour, baking soda, cinnamon, ginger, and salt in a large bowl. Set aside.

3. Mix the eggs, brown sugar, applesauce, honey, oil, orange zest, orange juice, and vanilla until combined in a medium bowl. Add the carrots and apple and whisk again.

4. Mix the dry and wet ingredients with a spatula. Fold in the raisins, pecans, and coconut. Mix everything once again, just until well combined. Put the batter into the prepared muffin cups, filling them to the top.

5. Bake between 20 to 25 minutes, or until a wooden toothpick inserted into the middle of the center muffin comes out clean (switching racks halfway through if baking on 2 racks). Cool for 5 minutes in the tins, then transfers to a wire rack to cool for an additional 5 minutes. Cool completely before storing in containers.

Nutrition:

- Calories: 292
- Fat: 14g
- Carbohydrates: 42g
- Protein: 5g
- Sodium: 84mg

27. Bagels Made Healthy

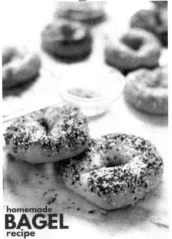

homemade BAGEL recipe

Preparation Time: 5 minutes
Cooking Time: 40 minutes
Servings: 8
Ingredients:

- 1 ½ c. warm water
- 1 ¼ c. bread flour
- 2 tbsps. Honey
- 2 c. whole wheat flour
- 2 tsp. Yeast
- 1 ½ tbsps. Olive oil
- 1 tbsp. vinegar

Directions:

1. In a bread machine, mix all ingredients, and then process on dough cycle. Once done, create 8 pieces shaped like a flattened ball. Create a donut shape using your thumb to make a hole at the center of each ball.

2. Place donut-shaped dough on a greased baking sheet, then cover and let it rise about ½ hour. Prepare about 2 inches of water to boil in a large pan.

3. In boiling water, drop one at a time the bagels and boil for 1 minute, then turn them once. Remove them and return them to the baking sheet and bake at 350oF for about 20 to 25 minutes until golden brown.

Nutrition:

- Calories: 228
- Fat: 3.7 g
- Carbs: 41.8 g
- Protein: 6.9 g
- Sugars: 0 g
- Sodium: 15 mg

28. Cereal with Cranberry-Orange Twist

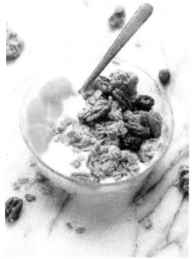

Preparation Time: 5 minutes
Cooking Time: 0 minutes
Servings: 1
Ingredients:

- ½ c. water
- ½ c. orange juice
- 1/3 c. oat bran
- ¼ c. dried cranberries
- Sugar
- Milk

Directions:

1. In a bowl, combine all ingredients. For about 2 minutes, microwave the bowl, then serve with sugar and milk. Enjoy!

Nutrition:

- Calories: 220

- Fat: 2.4 g
- Carbs: 43.5 g
- Protein: 6.2 g
- Sugars: 8 g
- Sodium: 1 mg

29. No Cook Overnight Oats

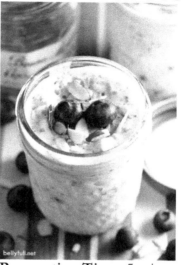

Preparation Time: 5 minutes
Cooking Time: 0 minutes
Servings: 1
Ingredients:

- 1 ½ c. low-fat milk
- 5 whole almond pieces
- 1 tsp. chia seeds
- 2 tbsps. Oats
- 1 tsp. sunflower seeds
- 1 tbsp. Craisins

Directions:

1. In a jar or mason bottle with a cap, mix all ingredients. Refrigerate overnight. Enjoy for breakfast.

Nutrition:

- Calories: 271
- Fat: 9.8 g
- Carbs: 35.4 g
- Protein: 16.7 g

- Sugars: 9
- Sodium: 103 mg

30. Avocado Cup with Egg

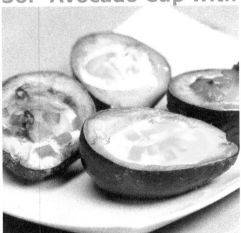

Preparation Time: 5 minutes
Cooking Time: 0 minutes
Servings: 4
Ingredients:
- 4 tsp. parmesan cheese
- 1 chopped stalk scallion
- 4 dashes pepper
- 4 dashes paprika
- 2 ripe avocados
- 4 medium eggs

Directions:

1. Preheat oven to 375F. Slice avocadoes in half and discard the seed. Slice the rounded portions of the avocado to make it level and sit well on a baking sheet.

2. Place avocadoes on a baking sheet and crack one egg in each hole of the avocado. Season each egg evenly with pepper and paprika. Bake for 25 minutes or until eggs are cooked to your liking. Serve with a sprinkle of parmesan.

Nutrition:
- Calories: 206
- Fat: 15.4 g
- Carbs: 11.3 g
- Protein: 8.5 g
- Sugars: 0.4 g
- Sodium: 21 mg

31. Gnocchi with Tomato Basil Sauce

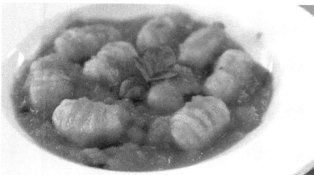

Preparation Time: 15 minutes
Cooking Time: 25 minutes
Servings: 6
Ingredients:

- 2 tablespoons olive oil
- ½ yellow onion, peeled and diced
- 3 cloves garlic, peeled and minced
- 1 (32-ounce) can no-salt-added crushed San Marzano tomatoes
- ¼ cup fresh basil leaves
- 2 teaspoons Italian seasoning
- ½ teaspoon kosher or sea salt
- 1 teaspoon granulated sugar
- ½ teaspoon ground black pepper
- 1/8 teaspoon crushed red pepper flakes
- 1 tablespoon heavy cream (optional)
- 12 ounces gnocchi
- ¼ cup freshly grated Parmesan cheese

Directions:
1. Heat the olive oil in a Dutch oven or stockpot over medium heat. Add the onion and sauté for 5 to 6 minutes until soft. Stir in the garlic and stir until fragrant, 30 to 60 seconds. Then stir in the tomatoes, basil, Italian seasoning, salt, sugar, black pepper, and crushed red pepper flakes.
2. Bring to a simmer for 15 minutes. Stir in the heavy cream, if desired. For a smooth, puréed sauce, use an immersion blender or transfer sauce to a blender and purée until smooth. Taste and adjust the seasoning if necessary.
3. While the sauce simmers, cook the gnocchi according to the package instructions, remove with a slotted spoon, and transfer to 6 bowls. Pour the sauce over the gnocchi and top with the Parmesan cheese.

Nutrition:
- Calories: 287
- Fat: 7g
- Sodium: 527mg
- Carbohydrate: 41g
- Protein: 10g

32. Creamy Pumpkin Pasta

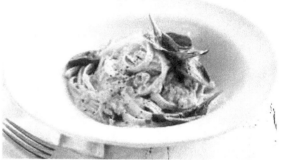

Preparation Time: 15 minutes
Cooking Time: 30 minutes
Servings: 6
Ingredients:

- 1-pound whole-grain linguine
- 1 tablespoon olive oil
- 3 garlic cloves, peeled and minced
- 2 tablespoons chopped fresh sage
- 1½ cups pumpkin purée
- 1 cup unsalted vegetable stock
- ½ cup low-fat evaporated milk
- ¾ teaspoon kosher or sea salt
- ½ teaspoon ground black pepper
- ½ teaspoon ground nutmeg
- ¼ teaspoon ground cayenne pepper

- ½ cup freshly grated Parmesan cheese, divided

Directions:
1. Cook the whole-grain linguine in a large pot of boiled water. Reserve ½ cup of pasta water and drain the rest. Set the pasta aside.
2. Heat olive oil over medium heat in a large skillet. Add the garlic and sage and sauté for 1 to 2 minutes until soft and fragrant. Whisk in the pumpkin purée, stock, milk, and reserved pasta water and simmer for 4 to 5 minutes, until thickened.
3. Whisk in the salt, black pepper, nutmeg, and cayenne pepper and half of the Parmesan cheese. Stir in the cooked whole-grain linguine. Evenly divide the pasta among 6 bowls and top with the remaining Parmesan cheese.

Nutrition:
- Calories: 381
- Fat: 8g
- Sodium: 175mg
- Carbohydrate: 63g
- Protein: 15g

33. Salmon Cakes with Bell Pepper Plus Lemon Yogurt

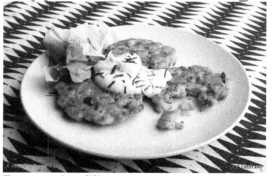

Preparation Time: 15 minutes
Cooking Time: 15 minutes
Servings: 4
Ingredients:

- ¼ cup whole-wheat bread crumbs
- ¼ cup mayonnaise
- 1 large egg, beaten
- 1 tablespoon chives, chopped
- 1 tablespoon fresh parsley, chopped
- Zest of 1 lemon
- ¾ teaspoon kosher salt, divided
- ¼ teaspoon freshly ground black pepper
- 2 (5- to 6-ounce) cans no-salt boneless/skinless salmon, drained and finely flaked
- ½ bell pepper, diced small
- 2 tablespoons extra-virgin olive oil, divided
- 1 cup plain Greek yogurt
- Juice of 1 lemon

Directions:
1. Mix the bread crumbs, mayonnaise, egg, chives, parsley, lemon zest, ½ teaspoon of salt, and black pepper in a large bowl. Add the salmon and the bell pepper and stir gently until well combined. Shape the mixture into 8 patties.
2. Heat 1 tablespoon of olive oil in a large skillet over medium-high heat. Cook half the cakes until the bottoms are golden brown, 4 to 5 minutes. Adjust the heat to medium if the bottoms start to burn.
3. Flip the cakes and cook until golden brown, an additional 4 to 5 minutes. Repeat the process with the rest of the 1 tablespoon olive oil and the rest of the cakes.
4. Mix the yogurt, lemon juice, and the remaining ¼ teaspoon salt in a small bowl. Serve with the salmon cakes.

Nutrition:
- Calories: 330
- Fat: 23g
- Sodium: 385mg
- Carbohydrates: 9g

- Protein: 21g

34. Steamed Fish Mediterranean Style

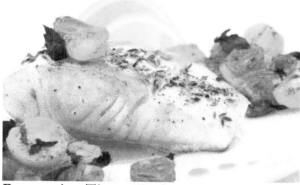

Preparation Time: 15 minutes
Cooking Time: 15 minutes
Servings: 4
Ingredients:

- Pepper to taste
- 1 clove garlic, smashed
- 2 tsp olive oil
- 1 bunch fresh thyme
- 2 tbsp pickled capers
- 1 cup black salt-cured olives
- 1-lb cherry tomatoes halved
- 1 ½-lbs. cod filets

Directions:

1. In a heat-proof dish that fits inside a saucepan, layer half of the halved cherry tomatoes. Season with pepper.
2. Add filets on top of tomatoes and season with pepper. Drizzle oil. Sprinkle 3/4s of thyme on top and the smashed garlic.
3. Cover top of fish with remaining cherry tomatoes, then place the dish on the trivet. Cover it with foil, then steam for 15 minutes. Serve and enjoy.

Nutrition:

- Calories: 263.2
- Carbs: 21.8g

- Protein: 27.8g
- Fats: 7.2g
- Sodium: 264mg

35. Steamed Veggie and Lemon Pepper Salmon

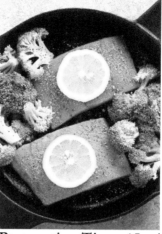

Preparation Time: 15 minutes
Cooking Time: 15 minutes
Servings: 4
Ingredients:

- 1 carrot, peeled and julienned
- 1 red bell pepper, julienned
- 1 zucchini, julienned
- ½ lemon, sliced thinly
- 1 tsp pepper
- ½ tsp salt
- 1/2-lb salmon filet with skin on
- A dash of tarragon

Directions:

1. In a heat-proof dish that fits inside a saucepan, add salmon with skin side down. Season with pepper. Add slices of lemon on top.
2. Place the julienned vegetables on top of salmon and season with tarragon. Cover top of fish with remaining cherry tomatoes and place dish on the trivet. Cover dish with foil. Cover pan and steam for 15 minutes. Serve and enjoy.

Nutrition:

- Calories: 216.2
- Carbs: 4.1g
- Protein: 35.1g
- Fats: 6.6g
- Sodium: 332mg

36. Steamed Fish with Scallions and Ginger

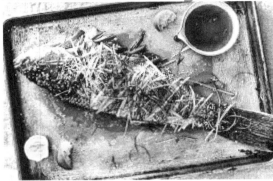

Preparation Time: 15 minutes
Cooking Time: 15 minutes
Servings: 3
Ingredients:

- ¼ cup chopped cilantro
- ¼ cup julienned scallions
- 2 tbsp julienned ginger
- 1 tbsp peanut oil
- 1-lb Tilapia filets
- 1 tsp garlic
- 1 tsp minced ginger
- 2 tbsp rice wine
- 1 tbsp low sodium soy sauce

Directions:

1. Mix garlic, minced ginger, rice wine, and soy sauce in a heat-proof dish that fits inside a saucepan. Add the Tilapia filet and marinate for half an hour while turning it over at the halftime.
2. Cover dish of fish with foil and place on a trivet. Cover pan and steam for 15 minutes. Serve and enjoy.

Nutrition:

- Calories: 219

- Carbs: 4.5g
- Protein: 31.8g
- Fats: 8.2g
- Sodium: 252mg

37. Rosemary Roasted Chicken

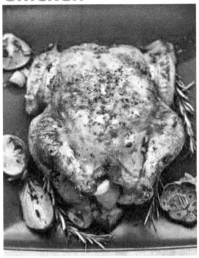

Preparation Time: 15 minutes
Cooking Time: 20 minutes
Servings: 8
Ingredients:

- 8 rosemary springs
- 1 minced garlic clove
- Black pepper
- 1 tbsp. chopped rosemary
- 1 chicken
- 1 tbsp. organic olive oil

Directions:

1. In a bowl, mix garlic with rosemary, rub the chicken with black pepper, the oil, and rosemary mix, place it inside a roasting pan, introduce inside the oven at 350F, and roast for sixty minutes and 20 minutes. Carve chicken, divide between plates and serve using a side dish. Enjoy!

Nutrition:

- Calories: 325

- Fat: 5 g
- Carbs: 15 g
- Protein: 14 g
- Sodium: 950 mg

38. Artichoke and Spinach Chicken

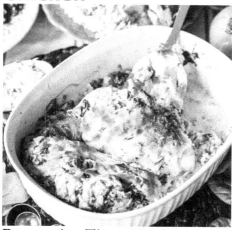

Preparation Time: 15 minutes
Cooking Time: 5 minutes
Servings: 4
Ingredients:

- 10 oz baby spinach
- ½ tsp. crushed red pepper flakes
- 14 oz. chopped artichoke hearts
- 28 oz. no-salt-added tomato sauce
- 2 tbsps. Essential olive oil
- 4 boneless and skinless chicken breasts

Directions:

1. Heat a pan with the oil over medium-high heat, add chicken and red pepper flakes and cook for 5 minutes on them. Add spinach, artichokes, and tomato sauce, toss, cook for ten minutes more, divide between plates and serve. Enjoy!

Nutrition:

- Calories: 212
- Fat: 3 g
- Carbs: 16 g

- Protein: 20 g
- Sugars: 5 g
- Sodium: 418 mg

39. Pumpkin and Black Beans Chicken

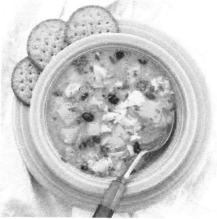

Preparation Time: 15 minutes
Cooking Time: 25 minutes
Servings: 4
Ingredients:

- 1 tbsp. essential olive oil
- 1 tbsp. Chopped cilantro
- 1 c. coconut milk
- 15 oz canned black beans, drained
- 1 lb. skinless and boneless chicken breasts
- 2 c. water
- ½ c. pumpkin flesh

Directions:

1. Heat a pan when using oil over medium-high heat, add the chicken and cook for 5 minutes. Add the river, milk, pumpkin, and black beans, toss, cover the pan, reduce heat to medium and cook for 20 mins. Add cilantro, toss, divide between plates and serve. Enjoy!

Nutrition:

- Calories: 254
- Fat: 6 g
- Carbs: 16 g

- Protein: 22 g
- Sodium: 92 mg

40. Chicken Thighs and Apples Mix

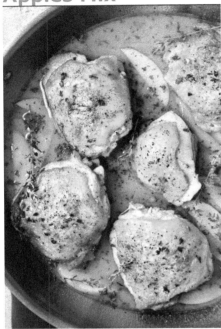

Preparation Time: 15 minutes
Cooking Time: 60 minutes
Servings: 4
Ingredients:

- 3 cored and sliced apples
- 1 tbsp apple cider vinegar treatment
- ¾ c. natural apple juice
- ¼ tsp. pepper and salt
- 1 tbsp. grated ginger
- 8 chicken thighs
- 3 tbsps. Chopped onion

Directions:

1.   In a bowl, mix chicken with salt, pepper, vinegar, onion, ginger, and apple juice, toss well, cover, keep in the fridge for ten minutes, transfer with a baking dish, and include apples. Introduce inside the oven at 400F for just 1 hour. Divide between plates and serve. Enjoy!

Nutrition:

- Calories: 214
- Fat: 3 g
- Carbs: 14 g
- Protein: 15 g
- Sodium: 405 mg

41. Healthy Chicken Orzo

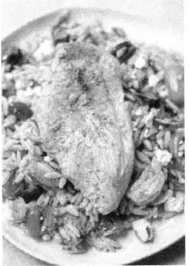

Preparation Time: 15 minutes
Cooking Time: 15 minutes
Servings: 4
Ingredients:

- 1 cup whole wheat orzo
- 1 lb. chicken breasts, sliced
- ½ tsp red pepper flakes
- ½ cup feta cheese, crumbled
- ½ tsp oregano
- 1 tbsp fresh parsley, chopped
- 1 tbsp fresh basil, chopped
- ¼ cup pine nuts
- 1 cup spinach, chopped
- ¼ cup white wine
- ½ cup olives, sliced
- 1 cup grape tomatoes, cut in half
- ½ tbsp garlic, minced

- 2 tbsp olive oil
- ½ tsp pepper
- ½ tsp salt

Directions:

1. Add water in a small saucepan and bring to a boil. Heat 1 tablespoon of olive oil in a pan over medium heat. Season chicken with pepper and salt and cook in the pan for 5-7 minutes on each side. Remove from pan and set aside.
2. Add orzo in boiling water and cook according to the packet directions. Heat the remaining olive oil in a pan on medium heat, then put garlic in the pan and sauté for a minute. Stir in white wine and cherry tomatoes and cook on high for 3 minutes.
3. Add cooked orzo, spices, spinach, pine nuts, and olives and stir until well combined. Add chicken on top of orzo and sprinkle with feta cheese. Serve and enjoy.

Nutrition:

- Calories: 518
- Fat: 27.7g
- Protein: 40.6g
- Carbs: 26.2g
- Sodium 121mg

42. Lemon Garlic Chicken

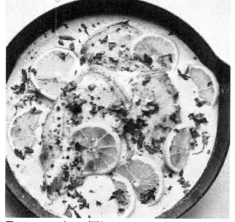

Preparation Time: 15 minutes
Cooking Time: 12 minutes
Servings: 3

Ingredients:

- 3 chicken breasts, cut into thin slices
- 2 lemon zest, grated
- ¼ cup olive oil
- 4 garlic cloves, minced
- Pepper
- Salt

Directions:

1. Heat olive oil in a pan over medium heat. Add garlic to the pan and sauté for 30 seconds. Put the chicken in the pan and sauté for 10 minutes. Add lemon zest and lemon juice and bring to boil. Remove from heat and season with pepper and salt. Serve and enjoy.

Nutrition:

- Calories: 439
- Fat: 27.8g
- Protein: 42.9g
- Carbs: 4.9g
- Sodium 306 mg

43. Simple Mediterranean Chicken

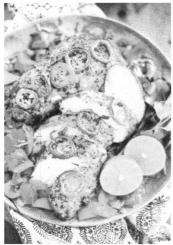

Preparation Time: 15 minutes
Cooking Time: 15 minutes
Servings: 12
Ingredients:

- 2 chicken breasts, skinless and boneless
- 1 ½ cup grape tomatoes, cut in half
- ½ cup olives
- 2 tbsp olive oil
- 1 tsp Italian seasoning
- ¼ tsp pepper
- ¼ tsp salt

Directions:

1. Season chicken with Italian seasoning, pepper, and salt. Heat olive oil in a pan over medium heat. Add season chicken to the pan and cook for 4-6 minutes on each side. Transfer chicken on a plate.
2. Put tomatoes plus olives in the pan and cook for 2-4 minutes. Pour olive and tomato mixture on top of the chicken and serve.

Nutrition:

- Calories: 468
- Fat: 29.4g
- Protein: 43.8g
- Carbs: 7.8g
- Sodium 410 mg

44. Roasted Chicken Thighs

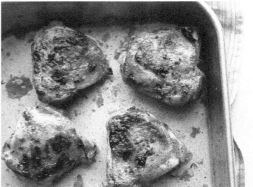

Preparation Time: 15 minutes
Cooking Time: 55 minutes
Servings: 4
Ingredients:

- 8 chicken thighs
- 3 tbsp fresh parsley, chopped
- 1 tsp dried oregano
- 6 garlic cloves, crushed
- ¼ cup capers, drained
- 10 oz roasted red peppers, sliced
- 2 cups grape tomatoes
- 1 ½ lbs. potatoes, cut into small chunks
- 4 tbsp olive oil
- Pepper
- Salt

Directions:

1. Warm oven to 200 C / 400 F. Season chicken with pepper and salt. Heat 2 tablespoons of olive oil in a pan over medium heat. Add chicken to the pan and sear until lightly golden brown from all the sides.
2. Transfer chicken onto a baking tray. Add tomato, potatoes, capers, oregano, garlic, and red peppers around the chicken. Season with pepper and salt and drizzle with remaining olive oil. Bake in the preheated oven for 45-55 minutes. Garnish with parsley and serve.

Nutrition:
- Calories: 848
- Fat: 29.1g
- Protein: 91.3g
- Carbs: 45.2g
- Sodium 110 mg

45. Mediterranean Turkey Breast

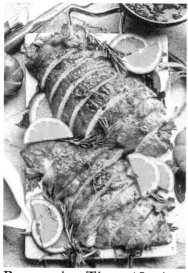

Preparation Time: 15 minutes
Cooking Time: 4 minutes & 30 minutes
Servings: 6
Ingredients:
- 4 lbs. turkey breast
- 3 tbsp flour
- ¾ cup chicken stock
- 4 garlic cloves, chopped
- 1 tsp dried oregano
- ½ fresh lemon juice
- ½ cup sun-dried tomatoes, chopped
- ½ cup olives, chopped
- 1 onion, chopped
- ¼ tsp pepper
- ½ tsp salt

Directions:

1. Add turkey breast, garlic, oregano, lemon juice, sun-dried tomatoes, olives, onion, pepper, and salt to the slow cooker. Add half stock. Cook on high for 4 hours.
2. Whisk remaining stock and flour in a small bowl and add to the slow cooker. Cover and cook for 30 minutes more. Serve and enjoy.

Nutrition:
- Calories: 537
- Fat: 9.7g
- Protein: 79.1g
- Carbs: 29.6g
- Sodium 330 mg

46. Thai Chicken Thighs

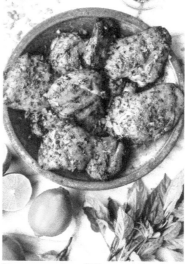

Preparation Time: 15 minutes
Cooking Time: 1 hour & 5 minutes
Servings: 6
Ingredients:
- ½ c. Thai chili sauce
- 1 chopped green onions bunch
- 4 lbs. chicken thighs

Directions:

1. Heat a pan over medium-high heat. Add chicken thighs, brown them for 5 minutes on both sides. Transfer to some baking dish, then add chili sauce and green onions and toss.

2. Introduce into the oven and bake at 400F for 60 minutes. Divide everything between plates and serve. Enjoy!

Nutrition:

- Calories: 220
- Fat: 4 g
- Carbs: 12 g
- Protein: 10 g
- Sodium: 870 mg

47. Falling "Off" The Bone Chicken

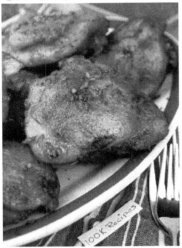

Preparation Time: 15 minutes
Cooking Time: 40 minutes
Servings: 4
Ingredients:

- 6 peeled garlic cloves
- 1 tbsp. organic extra virgin coconut oil
- 2 tbsps. Lemon juice
- 1 ½ c. pacific organic bone chicken broth
- ¼ tsp freshly ground black pepper
- ½ tsp. sea flavored vinegar
- 1 whole organic chicken piece
- 1 tsp. paprika
- 1 tsp. dried thyme

Directions:

1. Take a small bowl and toss in the thyme, paprika, pepper, and flavored vinegar and mix them. Use the mixture to season the chicken properly. Pour down the oil in your instant pot and heat it to shimmering; toss in the chicken with breast downward and let it cook for about 6-7 minutes

2. After 7 minutes, flip over the chicken, pour down the broth, garlic cloves, and lemon juice. Cook for 25 minutes on a high setting. Remove the dish from the cooker and let it stand for about 5 minutes before serving.

Nutrition:

- Calories: 664
- Fat: 44 g
- Carbs: 44 g
- Protein: 27 g
- Sugars: 0.1 g
- Sodium: 800 mg

48. Feisty Chicken Porridge

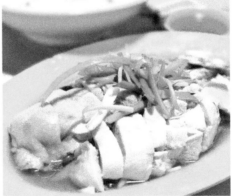

Preparation Time: 15 minutes
Cooking Time: 30 minutes
Servings: 4
Ingredients:

- 1 ½ c. fresh ginger
- 1 lb. cooked chicken legs
- Green onions
- Toasted cashew nuts
- 5 c. chicken broth

- 1 cup jasmine rice
- 4 c. water

Directions:

1. Place the rice in your fridge and allow it to chill 1 hour before cooking. Take the rice out and add them to your Instant Pot. Pour broth and water. Lock up the lid and cook on Porridge mode.

2. Separate the meat from the chicken legs and add the meat to your soup. Stir well over sauté mode. Season with a bit of flavored vinegar and enjoy with a garnish of nuts and onion

Nutrition:

- Calories: 206
- Fat: 8 g
- Carbs: 8 g
- Protein: 23 g
- Sugars: 0 g
- Sodium: 950 mg

49. Steamed Tilapia with Green Chutney

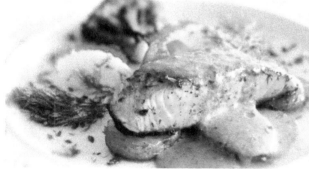

Preparation Time: 15 minutes
Cooking Time: 10 minutes
Servings: 3
Ingredients:

- 1-pound tilapia fillets, divided into 3
- ½ cup green commercial chutney

Directions:

1. Cut 3 pieces of 15-inch length foil. In one foil, place one filet in the middle and 1/3 of chutney. Fold over the foil and seal the filet inside. Repeat the process for the remaining fish. Put the packet on the trivet. Steam for 10 minutes. Serve and enjoy.

Nutrition:

- Calories: 151.5
- Carbs: 1.1g
- Protein: 30.7g
- Fats: 2.7g
- Sodium: 79mg

50. Creamy Haddock with Kale

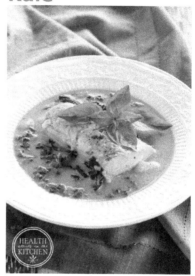

Preparation Time: 15 minutes
Cooking Time: 10 minutes
Servings: 5
Ingredients:

- 1 tbsp olive oil
- 1 onion, chopped
- 2 cloves of garlic, minced
- 2 cups chicken broth
- 1 teaspoon crushed red pepper flakes
- 1-pound wild Haddock fillets
- ½ cup heavy cream
- 1 tablespoon basil
- 1 cup kale leaves, chopped

- Pepper to taste

Directions:

1. Place a pot on medium-high fire for 3 minutes. Put oil, then sauté the onion and garlic for 5 minutes. Put the rest of the ingredients, except for basil, and mix well. Boil on lower fire for 5 minutes. Serve with a sprinkle of basil.

Nutrition:

- Calories: 130.5
- Carbs: 5.5g
- Protein: 35.7g
- Fats: 14.5g
- Sodium: 278mg

51. Loaded Baked Sweet Potatoes

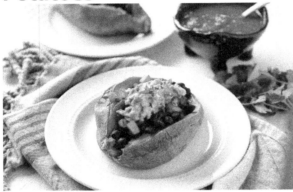

Preparation Time: 15 minutes
Cooking Time: 20 minutes
Servings: 4
Ingredients:

- 4 sweet potatoes
- ½ cup nonfat or low-fat plain Greek yogurt
- Freshly ground black pepper
- 1 teaspoon olive oil
- 1 red bell pepper, cored and diced
- ½ red onion, diced
- 1 teaspoon ground cumin

- 1 (15-ounce) can chickpeas, drained and rinsed

Directions:

1. Prick the potatoes using a fork and cook on your microwave's potato setting until potatoes are soft and cooked through, about 8 to 10 minutes for 4 potatoes. If you don't have a microwave, bake at 400°F for about 45 minutes.
2. Combine the yogurt and black pepper in a small bowl and mix well. Heat the oil in a medium pot over medium heat. Add bell pepper, onion, cumin, and additional black pepper to taste.
3. Add the chickpeas, stir to combine, and heat through about 5 minutes. Slice the potatoes lengthwise down the middle and top each half with a portion of the bean mixture followed by 1 to 2 tablespoons of the yogurt. Serve immediately.

Nutrition:

- Calories: 264
- Fat: 2g
- Sodium: 124mg
- Carbohydrate: 51g
- Protein: 11g

52. White Beans with Spinach and Pan-Roasted Tomatoes

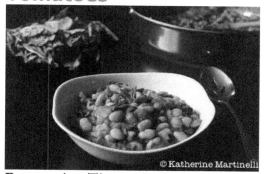
© Katherine Martinelli

Preparation Time: 15 minutes
Cooking Time: 10 minutes
Servings: 2
Ingredients:

- 1 tablespoon olive oil
- 4 small plum tomatoes, halved lengthwise
- 10 ounces frozen spinach, defrosted and squeezed of excess water
- 2 garlic cloves, thinly sliced
- 2 tablespoons water
- ¼ teaspoon freshly ground black pepper
- 1 can white beans, drained
- Juice of 1 lemon

Directions:
1. Heat the oil in a large skillet over medium-high heat. Put the tomatoes, cut-side down, and cook for 3 to 5 minutes; turn and cook for 1 minute more. Transfer to a plate.
2. Reduce heat to medium and add the spinach, garlic, water, and pepper to the skillet. Cook, tossing until the spinach is heated through, 2 to 3 minutes.
3. Return the tomatoes to the skillet, put the white beans and lemon juice, and toss until heated through 1 to 2 minutes.

Nutrition:
- Calories: 293
- Fat: 9g
- Sodium: 267mg
- Carbohydrate: 43g
- Protein: 15g

53. Black-Eyed Peas and Greens Power Salad

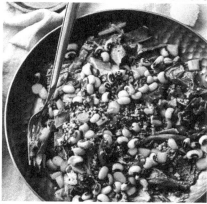

Preparation Time: 15 minutes
Cooking Time: 6 minutes
Servings: 2
Ingredients:

- 1 tablespoon olive oil
- 3 cups purple cabbage, chopped
- 5 cups baby spinach
- 1 cup shredded carrots
- 1 can black-eyed peas, drained
- Juice of ½ lemon
- Salt
- Freshly ground black pepper

Directions:
1. In a medium pan, add the oil and cabbage and sauté for 1 to 2 minutes on medium heat. Add in your spinach, cover for 3 to 4 minutes on medium heat, until greens are wilted. Remove from the heat and add to a large bowl.
2. Add in the carrots, black-eyed peas, and a splash of lemon juice. Season with salt and pepper, if desired. Toss and serve.

Nutrition:

- Calories: 320
- Fat: 9g
- Sodium: 351mg
- Potassium: 544mg
- Carbohydrate: 49g
- Protein: 16g

54. Butternut-Squash Macaroni and Cheese

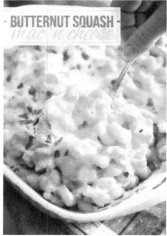

Preparation Time: 15 minutes
Cooking Time: 20 minutes
Servings: 2
Ingredients:

- 1 cup whole-wheat ziti macaroni
- 2 cups peeled and cubed butternut squash
- 1 cup nonfat or low-fat milk, divided
- Freshly ground black pepper
- 1 teaspoon Dijon mustard
- 1 tablespoon olive oil
- ¼ cup shredded low-fat cheddar cheese

Directions:

1. Cook the pasta al dente. Put the butternut squash plus ½ cup milk in a medium saucepan and place over medium-high heat. Season with black pepper. Bring it to a simmer. Lower the heat, then cook until fork-tender, 8 to 10 minutes.

2. To a blender, add squash and Dijon mustard. Purée until smooth. Meanwhile, place a large sauté pan over medium heat and add olive oil. Add the squash purée and the remaining ½ cup of milk. Simmer for 5 minutes. Add the cheese and stir to combine.

3. Add the pasta to the sauté pan and stir to combine. Serve immediately.

Nutrition:

- Calories: 373
- Fat: 10g
- Sodium: 193mg
- Carbohydrate: 59g
- Protein: 14g

55. Coconut Curry Sea Bass

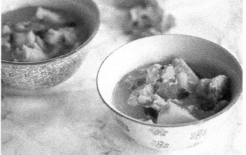

Preparation Time: 15 minutes
Cooking Time: 15 minutes
Servings: 3
Ingredients:

- 1 can coconut milk
- Juice of 1 lime, freshly squeezed
- 1 tablespoon red curry paste
- 1 teaspoon coconut aminos
- 1 teaspoon honey
- 2 teaspoons sriracha
- 2 cloves of garlic, minced
- 1 teaspoon ground turmeric
- 1 tablespoon curry powder
- ¼ cup fresh cilantro
- Pepper

Directions:

1. Place a heavy-bottomed pot on a medium-high fire. Mix in all ingredients, then simmer on lower fire to a simmer and simmer for 5 minutes. Serve and enjoy.

Nutrition:
- Calories: 241.8
- Carbs: 12.8g
- Protein: 3.1g
- Fats: 19.8g
- Sodium: 19mg

56. Halibut in Parchment with Zucchini, Shallots, and Herbs

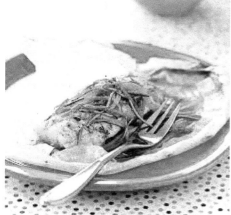

Preparation Time: 15 minutes
Cooking Time: 15 minutes
Servings: 4
Ingredients:
- ½ cup zucchini, diced small
- 1 shallot, minced
- 4 (5-ounce) halibut fillets (about 1 inch thick)
- 4 teaspoons extra-virgin olive oil
- ¼ teaspoon kosher salt
- 1/8 teaspoon freshly ground black pepper
- 1 lemon, sliced into 1/8 -inch-thick rounds
- 8 sprigs of thyme

Directions:
1. Preheat the oven to 450°F. Combine the zucchini and shallots in a medium bowl. Cut 4 (15-by-24-inch) pieces of parchment paper. Fold each sheet in half horizontally.
2. Draw a large half heart on one side of each folded sheet, with the fold along the heart center. Cut out the heart, open the parchment, and lay it flat.
3. Place a fillet near the center of each parchment heart. Drizzle 1 teaspoon olive oil on each fillet. Sprinkle with salt and pepper. Top each fillet with lemon slices and 2 sprigs of thyme. Sprinkle each fillet with one-quarter of the zucchini and shallot mixture. Fold the parchment over.
4. Starting at the top, fold the parchment edges over, and continue all the way around to make a packet. Twist the end tightly to secure. Arrange the 4 packets on a baking sheet. Bake for about 15 minutes. Place on plates; cut open. Serve immediately.

Nutrition:
- Calories: 190
- Fat: 7g
- Sodium: 170mg
- Carbohydrates: 5g
- Protein: 27g

57. Flounder with Tomatoes and Basil

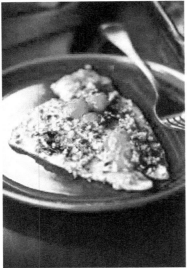

Preparation Time: 15 minutes
Cooking Time: 20 minutes
Servings: 4
Ingredients:

- 1-pound cherry tomatoes
- 4 garlic cloves, sliced
- 2 tablespoons extra-virgin olive oil
- 2 tablespoons lemon juice
- 2 tablespoons basil, cut into ribbons
- ½ teaspoon kosher salt
- ¼ teaspoon freshly ground black pepper
- 4 (5- to 6-ounce) flounder fillets

Directions:

1. Preheat the oven to 425°F.
2. Mix the tomatoes, garlic, olive oil, lemon juice, basil, salt, and black pepper in a baking dish. Bake for 5 minutes.
3. Remove, then arrange the flounder on top of the tomato mixture. Bake until the fish is opaque and begins to flake, about 10 to 15 minutes, depending on thickness.

Nutrition:

- Calories: 215
- Fat: 9g
- Sodium: 261mg
- Carbohydrates: 6g
- Protein: 28g

58. Grilled Mahi-Mahi with Artichoke Caponata

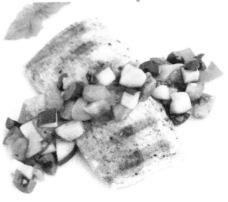

Preparation Time: 15 minutes
Cooking Time: 30 minutes
Servings: 4
Ingredients:

- 2 tablespoons extra-virgin olive oil
- 2 celery stalks, diced
- 1 onion, diced
- 2 garlic cloves, minced
- ½ cup cherry tomatoes, chopped
- ¼ cup white wine
- 2 tablespoons white wine vinegar
- 1 can artichoke hearts, drained and chopped
- ¼ cup green olives, pitted and chopped
- 1 tablespoon capers, chopped
- ¼ teaspoon red pepper flakes
- 2 tablespoons fresh basil, chopped
- 4 (5- to 6-ounces each) skinless mahi-mahi fillets
- ½ teaspoon kosher salt
- ¼ teaspoon freshly ground black pepper

- Olive oil cooking spray

Directions:

1. Heat olive oil in a skillet over medium heat, then put the celery and onion and sauté for 4 to 5 minutes. Add the garlic and sauté for 30 seconds. Add the tomatoes and cook for 2 to 3 minutes. Add the wine and vinegar to deglaze the pan, increasing the heat to medium-high.
2. Add the artichokes, olives, capers, and red pepper flakes and simmer, reducing the liquid by half, about 10 minutes. Mix in the basil.
3. Season the mahi-mahi with salt and pepper. Heat a grill skillet or grill pan over medium-high heat and coat with olive oil cooking spray. Add the fish and cook for 4 to 5 minutes per side. Serve topped with the artichoke caponata.

Nutrition:

- Calories: 245
- Fat: 9g
- Sodium: 570mg
- Carbohydrates: 10g
- Protein: 28g

59. Cod and Cauliflower Chowder

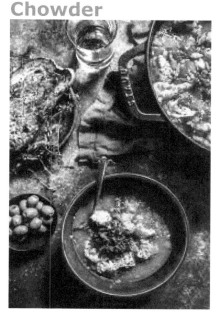

Preparation Time: 15 minutes
Cooking Time: 40 minutes
Servings: 4
Ingredients:

- 2 tablespoons extra-virgin olive oil
- 1 leek, sliced thinly
- 4 garlic cloves, sliced
- 1 medium head cauliflower, coarsely chopped
- 1 teaspoon kosher salt
- ¼ teaspoon freshly ground black pepper
- 2 pints cherry tomatoes
- 2 cups no-salt-added vegetable stock
- ¼ cup green olives, pitted and chopped
- 1 to 1½ pounds cod
- ¼ cup fresh parsley, minced

Directions:

1. Heat the olive oil in a Dutch oven or large pot over medium heat. Add the leek and sauté until lightly golden brown, about 5 minutes.
2. Add the garlic and sauté for 30 seconds. Add the cauliflower, salt, and black pepper and sauté for 2 to 3 minutes.
3. Add the tomatoes and vegetable stock, increase the heat to high and boil, then turn the heat to low and simmer for 10 minutes.
4. Add the olives and mix. Add the fish, cover, and simmer for 20 minutes or until the fish is opaque and flakes easily. Gently mix in the parsley.

Nutrition:

- Calories: 270
- Fat: 9g
- Sodium: 545mg
- Potassium: 1475mg
- Carbohydrates: 19g
- Protein: 30g

60. Sardine Bruschetta with Fennel and Lemon Crema

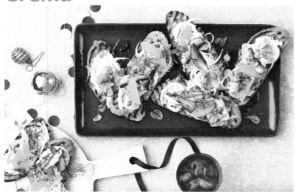

Preparation Time: 15 minutes
Cooking Time: 0 minutes
Servings: 4
Ingredients:

- 1/3 cup plain Greek yogurt
- 2 tablespoons mayonnaise
- 2 tablespoons lemon juice, divided
- 2 teaspoons lemon zest
- ¾ teaspoon kosher salt, divided
- 1 fennel bulb, cored and thinly sliced
- ¼ cup parsley, chopped, plus more for garnish
- ¼ cup fresh mint, chopped2 teaspoons extra-virgin olive oil
- 1/8 teaspoon freshly ground black pepper
- 8 slices multigrain bread, toasted
- 2 (4.4-ounce) cans of smoked sardines

Directions:
1. Mix the yogurt, mayonnaise, 1 tablespoon of lemon juice, the lemon zest, and ¼ teaspoon of salt in a small bowl.
2. Mix the remaining ½ teaspoon salt, the remaining 1 tablespoon lemon juice, the fennel, parsley, mint, olive oil, and black pepper in a separate small bowl.

3. Spoon 1 tablespoons of the yogurt mixture on each piece of toast. Divide the fennel mixture evenly on top of the yogurt mixture. Divide the sardines among the toasts, placing them on top of the fennel mixture. Garnish with more herbs, if desired.

Nutrition:
- Calories: 400
- Fat: 16g
- Sodium: 565mg
- Carbohydrates: 51g
- Protein: 16g

61. Mexican-Style Potato Casserole

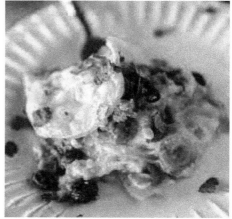

Preparation Time: 15 minutes
Cooking Time: 60 minutes
Servings: 8
Ingredients:

- Cooking spray
- 2 tablespoons canola oil
- ½ yellow onion, peeled and diced
- 4 garlic cloves, peeled and minced
- 2 tablespoons all-purpose flour
- 1¼ cups milk
- 1 tablespoon chili powder
- ½ tablespoon ground cumin
- 1 teaspoon kosher salt or sea salt

- ½ teaspoon ground black pepper
- ¼ teaspoon ground cayenne pepper
- 1½ cups shredded Mexican-style cheese, divided
- 1 (4-ounce) can green chilis, drained
- 1½ pounds baby Yukon Gold or red potatoes, thinly sliced
- 1 red bell pepper, thinly sliced

Directions:

1. Preheat the oven to 400°F. Oiled a 9-by-13-inch baking dish with cooking spray. In a large saucepan, warm canola oil on medium heat. Add the onion and sauté for 4 to 5 minutes until soft. Mix in the garlic, then cook until fragrant, 30 to 60 seconds.

2. Mix in the flour, then put in the milk while whisking. Slow simmer for about 5 minutes until thickened. Whisk in the chili powder, cumin, salt, black pepper, and cayenne pepper.

3. Remove from the heat and whisk in half of the shredded cheese and the green chilis. Taste and adjust the seasoning if necessary. Line up one-third of the sliced potatoes and sliced bell pepper in the baking dish and top with a quarter of the remaining shredded cheese.

4. Repeat with 2 more layers. Pour the cheese sauce over the top and sprinkle with the remaining shredded cheese. Cover it with aluminum foil and bake for 45 to 50 minutes until the potatoes are tender.

5. Remove the foil and bake again for 5 to 10 minutes until the topping is slightly browned. Let cool for 20 minutes before slicing into 8 pieces. Serve.

Nutrition:

- Calories: 195
- Fat: 10g
- Sodium: 487mg
- Carbohydrate: 19g
- Protein: 8g

62. Spicy Tofu Burrito Bowls with Cilantro Avocado Sauce

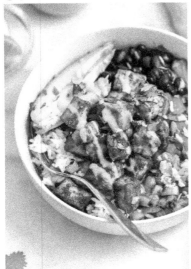

Preparation Time: 15 minutes
Cooking Time: 15 minutes
Servings: 4
Ingredients:
For the sauce:

- ¼ cup plain nonfat Greek yogurt
- ½ cup fresh cilantro leaves
- ½ ripe avocado, peeled
- Zest and juice of 1 lime
- 2 garlic cloves, peeled
- ¼ teaspoon kosher or sea salt
- 2 tablespoons water

For the burrito bowls:

- 1 (14-ounce) package extra-firm tofu
- 1 tablespoon canola oil
- 1 yellow or orange bell pepper, diced
- 2 tablespoons Taco Seasoning
- ¼ teaspoon kosher or sea salt
- 2 cups Fluffy Brown Rice
- 1 (15-ounce) can black beans, drained

Directions:

1. Place all the sauce ingredients in the bowl of a food processor or blender and purée until smooth. Taste and adjust the seasoning if necessary. Refrigerate until ready for use.
2. Put the tofu on your plate lined with a kitchen towel. Put another kitchen towel over the tofu and place a heavy pot on top, changing towels if they become soaked. Let it stand for 15 minutes to remove the moisture. Cut the tofu into 1-inch cubes.
3. Heat canola oil in a large skillet over medium heat. Add the tofu and bell pepper and sauté, breaking up the tofu into smaller pieces for 4 to 5 minutes. Stir in the taco seasoning, salt, and ¼ cup of water. Evenly divide the rice and black beans among 4 bowls. Top with the tofu/bell pepper mixture and top with the cilantro avocado sauce.

Nutrition:

- Calories: 383
- Fat: 13g
- Sodium: 438mg
- Carbohydrate: 48g
- Protein: 21g

63. Sweet Potato Cakes with Classic Guacamole

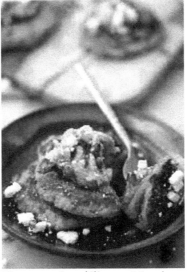

Preparation Time: 15 minutes

Cooking Time: 20 minutes
Servings: 4
Ingredients:
For the guacamole:

- 2 ripe avocados, peeled and pitted
- ½ jalapeño, seeded and finely minced
- ¼ red onion, peeled and finely diced
- ¼ cup fresh cilantro leaves, chopped
- Zest and juice of 1 lime
- ¼ teaspoon kosher or sea salt

For the cakes:

- 3 sweet potatoes, cooked and peeled
- ½ cup cooked black beans
- 1 large egg
- ½ cup panko bread crumbs
- 1 teaspoon ground cumin
- 1 teaspoon chili powder
- ½ teaspoon kosher or sea salt
- ¼ teaspoon ground black pepper
- 2 tablespoons canola oil

Directions:

1. Mash the avocado, then stir in the jalapeño, red onion, cilantro, lime zest and juice, and salt in a bowl. Taste and adjust the seasoning if necessary.
2. Put the cooked sweet potatoes plus black beans in a bowl and mash until a paste form. Stir in the egg, bread crumbs, cumin, chili powder, salt, and black pepper until combined.
3. Heat canola oil in a large skillet at medium heat. Form the sweet potato mixture into 4 patties, place them in the hot skillet, and cook for 3 to 4 minutes per side until browned and crispy. Serve the sweet potato cakes with guacamole on top.

Nutrition:

- Calories: 369
- Fat: 22g
- Sodium: 521mg
- Carbohydrate: 38g
- Protein: 8g

64. Chickpea Cauliflower Tikka Masala

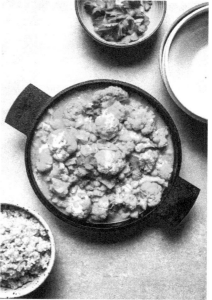

Preparation Time: 15 minutes
Cooking Time: 40 minutes
Servings: 6
Ingredients:

- 2 tablespoons olive oil
- 1 yellow onion, peeled and diced
- 4 garlic cloves, peeled and minced
- 1-inch piece fresh ginger, peeled and minced
- 2 tablespoons Garam Masala
- 1 teaspoon kosher or sea salt
- ½ teaspoon ground black pepper
- ¼ teaspoon ground cayenne pepper
- ½ small head cauliflower, small florets
- 2 (15-ounce) cans of no-salt-added chickpeas, rinsed and drained
- 1 (15-ounce) can no-salt-added petite diced tomatoes, drained
- 1½ cups unsalted vegetable broth
- ½ (15-ounce) can coconut milk

- Zest and juice of 1 lime
- ½ cup fresh cilantro leaves, chopped, divided
- 1½ cups cooked Fluffy Brown Rice, divided

Directions:

1. Heat olive oil over medium heat, then put the onion and sauté for 4 to 5 minutes in a large Dutch oven or stockpot. Stir in the garlic, ginger, garam masala, salt, black pepper, and cayenne pepper and toast for 30 to 60 seconds, until fragrant.

2. Stir in the cauliflower florets, chickpeas, diced tomatoes, and vegetable broth and increase to medium-high. Simmer for 15 minutes until the cauliflower is fork-tender.

3. Remove, then stir in the coconut milk, lime juice, lime zest, and half of the cilantro. Taste and adjust the seasoning if necessary. Serve over the rice and the remaining chopped cilantro.

Nutrition:

- Calories: 323
- Fat: 12g
- Sodium: 444mg
- Carbohydrate: 44g
- Protein: 11g

65. Vegetable Noodles with Bolognese

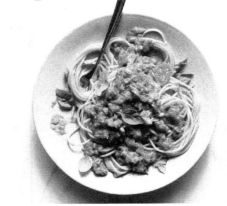

Preparation Time: 15 minutes

Cooking Time: 15 minutes
Servings: 4
Ingredients:

- 1.5 kg of small zucchini (e.g., green and yellow)
- 600g of carrots
- 1 onion
- 1 tbsp olive oil
- 250g of beef steak
- Pinch of Salt and pepper
- 2 tablespoons tomato paste
- 1 tbsp flour
- 1 teaspoon vegetable broth (instant)
- 40g pecorino or parmesan
- 1 small potty of basil

Directions:

1. Clean and peel zucchini and carrots and wash. Using a sharp, long knife, cut first into thin slices, then into long, fine strips. Clean or peel the soup greens, wash and cut into tiny cubes. Peel the onion and chop finely. Heat the Bolognese oil in a large pan. Fry hack in it crumbly. Season with salt and pepper.

2. Briefly sauté the prepared vegetable and onion cubes. Stir in tomato paste. Dust the flour, sweat briefly. Pour in 400 ml of water and stir in the vegetable stock. Boil everything, simmer for 7-8 minutes.

3. Meanwhile, cook the vegetable strips in plenty of salted water for 3-5 minutes. Drain, collecting some cooking water. Add the vegetable strips to the pan and mix well. If the sauce is not liquid enough, stir in some vegetable cooking water and season everything again.

4. Slicing cheese into fine shavings. Wash the basil, shake dry, peel off the leaves, and cut roughly. Arrange vegetable noodles, sprinkle with parmesan and basil.

Nutrition:

- Calories 269
- Fat 9.7g
- Protein 25.6g
- Sodium 253mg
- Carbohydrate 21.7g

66. Oregano Chicken Thighs

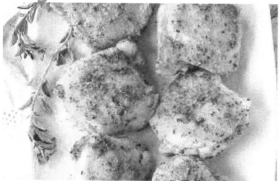

Preparation Time: 15 minutes
Cooking Time: 20 minutes
Servings: 6
Ingredients:

- 12 chicken thighs
- 1 tsp dried parsley
- ¼ tsp. pepper and salt.
- ½ c. extra virgin essential olive oil
- 4 minced garlic cloves
- 1 c. chopped oregano
- ¼ c. low-sodium veggie stock

Directions:

1. In your food processor, mix parsley with oregano, garlic, salt, pepper, and stock and pulse. Put chicken thighs for the bowl, add oregano paste, toss, cover, and then leave aside for the fridge for 10 minutes.
2. Heat the kitchen grill over medium heat, add chicken pieces, close the lid and cook for twenty or so minutes with them. Divide between plates and serve!

Nutrition:

- Calories: 254

- Fat: 3 g
- Carbs: 7 g
- Protein: 17 g
- Sugars: 0.9 g
- Sodium: 730 mg

67. Pesto Chicken Breasts with Summer Squash

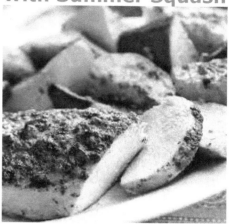

Preparation Time: 15 minutes
Cooking Time: 10 minutes
Servings: 4
Ingredients:

- 4 medium boneless, skinless chicken breast halves
- 1 tbsp. olive oil
- 2 tbsps. Homemade pesto
- 2 c. finely chopped zucchini
- 2 tbsps. Finely shredded Asiago

Directions:

1. Cook your chicken in hot oil on medium heat for 4 minutes in a large nonstick skillet. Flip the chicken, then put the zucchini.
2. Cook for 4 to 6 minutes more or until the chicken is tender and no longer pink (170 F), and squash is crisp-tender, stirring squash gently once or twice. Transfer chicken and squash to 4 dinner plates. Spread pesto over chicken; sprinkle with Asiago.

Nutrition:

- Calories: 230
- Fat: 9 g
- Carbs: 8 g
- Protein: 30 g
- Sodium: 578 mg

68. Chicken, Tomato and Green Beans

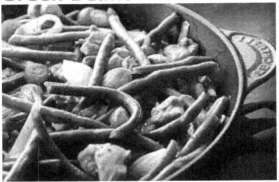

Preparation Time: 15 minutes
Cooking Time: 25 minutes
Servings: 4
Ingredients:

- 6 oz. low-sodium canned tomato paste
- 2 tbsps. Olive oil
- ¼ tsp. black pepper
- 2 lbs. trimmed green beans
- 2 tbsps. Chopped parsley
- 1 ½ lbs. boneless, skinless, and cubed chicken breasts
- 25 oz. no-salt-added canned tomato sauce

Directions:

1. Heat a pan with 50 % with the oil over medium heat, add chicken, stir, cover, cook for 5 minutes on both sides and transfer to a bowl. Heat inside the same pan while using rest through the oil over medium heat, add green beans, stir and cook for 10 minutes.
2. Return chicken for that pan, add black pepper, tomato sauce, tomato paste, and parsley, stir, cover, cook for 10 minutes more, divide between plates and serve. Enjoy!

Nutrition:

- Calories: 190
- Fat: 4 g
- Carbs: 12 g
- Protein: 9 g
- Sodium: 168 mg

69. Chicken Tortillas

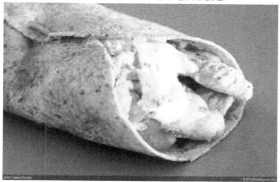

Preparation Time: 15 minutes
Cooking Time: 5 minutes
Servings: 4
Ingredients:

- 6 oz. boneless, skinless, and cooked chicken breasts
- Black pepper
- 1/3 c. fat-free yogurt
- 4 heated up whole-wheat tortillas
- 2 chopped tomatoes

Directions:

1. Heat a pan over medium heat, add one tortilla during those times, heat up, and hang them on the working surface. Spread yogurt on each tortilla, add chicken and tomatoes, roll, divide between plates and serve. Enjoy!

Nutrition:

- Calories: 190
- Fat: 2 g
- Carbs: 12 g
- Protein: 6 g
- Sodium: 300 mg

70. Harissa Bolognese with Vegetable Noodles

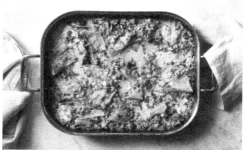

Preparation Time: 15 minutes
Cooking Time: 30 minutes
Servings: 4
Ingredients:

- 2 onions
- 1 clove of garlic
- 3-4 tbsp oil
- 400g ground beef
- Pinch salt, pepper, cinnamon
- 1 tsp Harissa (Arabic seasoning paste, tube)
- 1 tablespoon tomato paste
- 2 sweet potatoes
- 2 medium Zucchini
- 3 stems/basil
- 100g of feta

Directions:

1. Peel onions and garlic, finely dice. Heat 1 tbsp of oil in a wide saucepan. Fry hack in it crumbly. Fry onions and garlic for a short time. Season with salt, pepper, and ½ teaspoon cinnamon. Stir in harissa and tomato paste.
2. Add tomatoes and 200 ml of water, bring to the boil and simmer for about 15 minutes with occasional stirring. Peel sweet potatoes and zucchini or clean and wash. Cut vegetables into spaghetti with a spiral cutter.
3. Heat 2-3 tablespoons of oil in a large pan. Braise sweet potato spaghetti in it for about 3

minutes. Add the zucchini spaghetti and continue to simmer for 3-4 minutes while turning.

4. Season with salt and pepper. Wash the basil, shake dry and peel off the leaves. Garnish vegetable spaghetti and Bolognese on plates. Feta crumbles over. Sprinkle with basil.

Nutrition:

- Calories 452
- Fat 22.3g
- Protein 37.1g
- Sodium 253mg
- Carbohydrate 27.6g

71. Pesto Shrimp Pasta

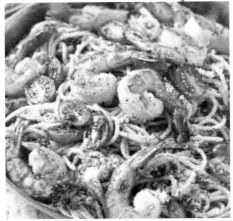

Preparation Time: 15 minutes
Cooking Time: 12 minutes
Servings: 4
Ingredients:

- 1/8 teaspoon freshly cracked pepper
- 1 cup dried orzo
- 4 tsp packaged pesto sauce mix
- 1 lemon, halved
- 1/8 teaspoon coarse salt
- 1-pound medium shrimp, thawed
- 1 medium zucchini, halved lengthwise and sliced
- 2 tablespoons olive oil, divided
- 1-ounce shaved Parmesan cheese

Directions:

1. Prepare orzo pasta concerning package directions. Drain; reserving ¼ cup of the pasta cooking water. Mix 1 teaspoon of the pesto mix into the kept cooking water and set aside.

2. Mix 3 teaspoons of the pesto mix plus 1 tablespoon of olive oil in a large plastic bag. Seal and shake to mix. Put the shrimp in the bag; seal and turn to coat. Set aside.

3. Sauté zucchini in a big skillet over moderate heat for 1 to 2 minutes, stirring repeatedly. Put the pesto-marinated shrimp in the skillet and cook for 5 minutes or until shrimp is dense.

4. Put the cooked pasta in the skillet with the zucchini and shrimp combination. Stir in the kept pasta water until absorbed, grating up any seasoning in the bottom of the pan. Season with pepper and salt. Squeeze the lemon over the pasta. Top with Parmesan, then serve.

Nutrition:

- Calories 361
- Fat 10.1 g
- Sodium 502 mg
- Carbohydrates 35.8 g
- Protein 31.6 g

72. Quick Shrimp Scampi

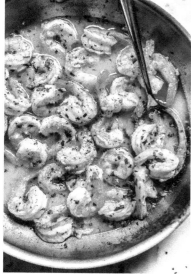

Preparation Time: 5 minutes
Cooking Time: 10 minutes
Servings: 4
Ingredients:

- 2 tablespoons olive oil
- ½ cup (120 ml) dry white wine
- 3 garlic cloves, minced
- 1 1/2 pound (680 g) large shrimp, peeled and stroked dry
- Large pinch of crushed red pepper flakes
- 1 lemon, zested, one half cut into slices
- 1/8 Salt
- 1/8 pepper
- 4 tbsp unsalted butter, slice into 4 pieces
- Large handful of fresh chopped flat-leaf parsley.

Directions:

1. In a large skillet, warm up the oil over moderate heat. Flavor the shrimp with salt plus pepper, then put them in the skillet in a single coating. Cook, without interruption, until the shrimp's bottoms begin to turn pink, about 1 minute after.

2. Turnover the shrimp and cook until almost cooked through, about 1 minute more. Keep the shrimp on a plate and set aside.

3. Adjust to medium, add the pepper flakes, garlic, and a little more oil if the pan seems dry; cook, repeatedly stirring until the garlic just begins to turn golden, about 1 minute. Add the wine, scraping up any burnt bits from the bottom of the pan, and simmer until most of the wine has vanished.

4. Mix in the butter, then season the sauce with lemon juice and salt from one lemon half. Add the cooked shrimp, the lemon zest, any juices accrued on the plate, and parsley and heave until the shrimp is warmed through, about 1 minute. Serve with lemon wedges if you wish.

Nutrition:

- Calories 316
- Fat 20.3 g
- Sodium 1039 mg
- Carbohydrates 4 g
- Protein 23.5 g

73. Poached Salmon with Creamy Piccata Sauce

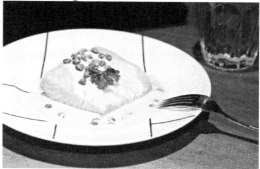

Preparation Time: 5 minutes
Cooking Time: 15 minutes
Servings: 4
Ingredients:

- 1-pound center-cut salmon fillet skinned and cut into 4 portions
- 2 tablespoons lemon juice

- 2 teaspoons extra-virgin olive oil
- ¼ cup reduced-fat sour cream
- 1 large shallot, minced
- 1 cup dry white wine, divided
- 1 tablespoon chopped fresh dill
- 4 teaspoons capers, rinsed
- ¼ teaspoon salt

Directions:

1. Place salmon in a wide skillet and add ½ cup wine and sufficient water to cover the salmon. Bring it to a boil over high-temperature heat. Simmer, turn the salmon over, cook for 5 minutes and then remove from the heat.

2. In the meantime, heat oil in a medium skillet over moderate heat. Add shallot and cook, stirring, until scented, about 30 seconds. Add the remaining ½ cup wine; boil until slightly condensed, about 1 minute.

3. Stir in lemon juice plus capers; cook 1 minute more. Remove, stir in sour cream and salt. Top the salmon with the sauce and relish it with dill before serving.

Nutrition:

- Calories 229
- Fat 8.3 g
- Sodium 286 mg
- Carbohydrates 3.7 g
- Protein 23.3 g

74. Chicken, Pasta and Snow Peas

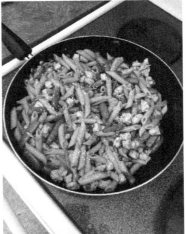

Preparation Time: 15 minutes
Cooking Time: 20 minutes
Servings: 2
Ingredients:

- 1-pound chicken breasts
- 2 ½ cups penne pasta
- 1 cup snow peas, trimmed and halved
- 1 teaspoon olive oil
- 1 standard jar Tomato and Basil pasta sauce
- Fresh ground pepper

Directions:

1. In a medium frying pan, heat the olive oil. Flavor the chicken breasts with salt and pepper. Cook the chicken breasts until cooked through (approximately 5 – 7 minutes each side).

2. Cook the pasta, as stated in the instruction of the package. Cook the snow peas with the pasta. Scoop 1 cup of the pasta water. Drain the pasta and peas, set them aside.

3. Once the chicken is cooked, slice diagonally. Return back the chicken to the frying pan. Add the pasta sauce. If the mixture seems dry, add some of the pasta water to the desired consistency. Heat, then divide into bowls. Serve immediately.

Nutrition:

- Calories - 140
- Protein - 34g
- Carbohydrates - 52g
- Fat - 17g
- Sodium - 118mg

75. Chicken with Noodles

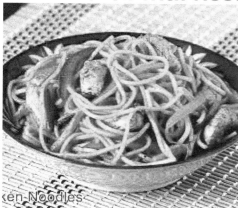

ken-Noodles

Preparation Time: 15 minutes
Cooking Time: 30 minutes
Servings: 6
Ingredients:

- 4 chicken breasts, skinless, boneless
- 1-pound pasta (angel hair, or linguine, or ramen)
- ½ teaspoon sesame oil
- 1 Tablespoon canola oil
- 2 Tablespoons chili paste
- 1 onion, diced
- 2 garlic cloves, chopped coarsely
- ½ cup of soy sauce
- ½ medium cabbage, sliced
- 2 carrots, chopped coarsely

Directions:

1. Cook your pasta in a large pot. Mix the canola oil, sesame oil, and chili paste and heat for 25 seconds in a large pot. Add the onion, cook for 2 minutes. Put the garlic and fry for 20 seconds. Add the chicken, cook on each side for 5 - 7 minutes, until cooked through.

2. Remove the mix from the pan, set aside. Add the cabbage, carrots, cook until the vegetables are tender. Pour everything back into the pan. Add the noodles. Pour into the soy sauce and combine thoroughly. Heat for 5 minutes. Serve immediately.

Nutrition:

- Calories - 110
- Protein - 30g
- Carbohydrates - 32g
- Sugars - 0.1g
- Fat - 18g
- Sodium - 121mg

76. Teriyaki Chicken Wings

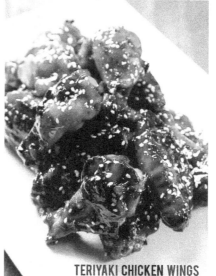

TERIYAKI CHICKEN WINGS

Preparation Time: 15 minutes
Cooking Time: 30 minutes
Servings: 6
Ingredients:

- 3 pounds of chicken wings (15 – 20)
- 1/3 cup lemon juice
- ¼ cup of soy sauce
- ¼ cup of vegetable oil
- 3 tablespoons chili sauce

- 1 garlic clove, finely chopped
- ¼ teaspoon fresh ground pepper
- ¼ teaspoon celery seed
- Dash liquid mustard

Directions:

1. Prepare the marinade. Combine lemon juice, soy sauce, chili sauce, oil, celery seed, garlic, pepper, and mustard. Stir well, set aside. Rinse and dry the chicken wings.

2. Pour marinade over the chicken wings. Coat thoroughly. Refrigerate for 2 hours. After 2 hours. Preheat the broiler in the oven. Drain off the excess sauce.

3. Place the wings on a cookie sheet with parchment paper. Broil on each side for 10 minutes. Serve immediately.

Nutrition:

- Calories - 96
- Protein - 15g
- Carbohydrates - 63g
- Fat - 15g
- Sodium- 145mg

77. Hot Chicken Wings

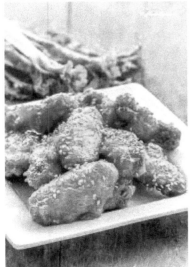

Preparation Time: 15 minutes

Cooking Time: 25 minutes
Servings: 4
Ingredients:

- 10 - 20 chicken wings
- ½ stick margarine
- 1 bottle Durkee hot sauce
- 2 Tablespoons honey
- 10 shakes Tabasco sauce
- 2 Tablespoons cayenne pepper

Directions:

1. Warm canola oil in a deep pot. Deep-fry the wings until cooked, approximately 20 minutes. Mix the hot sauce, honey, Tabasco, and cayenne pepper in a medium bowl. Mix well.

2. Place the cooked wings on paper towels. Drain the excess oil. Mix the chicken wings in the sauce until coated evenly.

Nutrition:

- Calories - 102
- Protein - 23g
- Carbohydrates - 55g
- Sugars - 0.1g
- Fat - 14g
- Sodium- 140mg

78. Peanut Vegetable Pad Thai

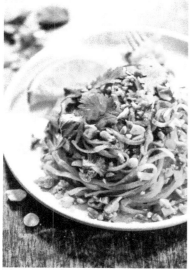

Preparation Time: 15 minutes
Cooking Time: 20 minutes
Servings: 6
Ingredients:

- 8 ounces brown rice noodles
- 1/3 cup natural peanut butter
- 3 tablespoons unsalted vegetable broth
- 1 tablespoon low-sodium soy sauce
- 2 tablespoons of rice wine vinegar
- 1 tablespoon honey
- 2 teaspoons sesame oil
- 1 teaspoon sriracha (optional)
- 1 tablespoon canola oil
- 1 red bell pepper, thinly sliced
- 1 zucchini, cut into matchsticks
- 2 large carrots, cut into matchsticks
- 3 large eggs, beaten
- ¾ teaspoon kosher or sea salt
- ½ cup unsalted peanuts, chopped
- ½ cup cilantro leaves, chopped

Directions:

1. Boil a large pot of water. Cook the rice noodles as stated in package directions. Mix the peanut butter, vegetable broth, soy sauce, rice wine vinegar, honey, sesame oil, and sriracha in a bowl. Set aside.

2. Heat canola oil over medium heat in a large nonstick skillet. Add the red bell pepper, zucchini, and carrots, and sauté for 2 to 3 minutes, until slightly soft. Stir in the eggs and fold with a spatula until scrambled. Add the cooked rice noodles, sauce, and salt. Toss to combine. Spoon into bowls and evenly top with the peanuts and cilantro.

Nutrition:

- Calories: 393
- Fat: 19g
- Sodium: 561mg
- Carbohydrate: 45g
- Protein: 13g

79. Tuscan-Style Tuna Salad

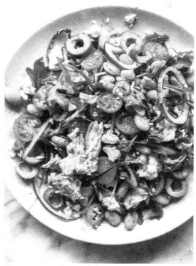

Preparation Time: 15 minutes
Cooking Time: 0 minutes
Servings: 4
Ingredients:

- 2 6-ounce cans chunk light tuna, drained.
- ¼ teaspoon salt
- 10 cherry tomatoes
- 2 tablespoons lemon juice
- 4 scallions, trimmed and sliced
- 2 tablespoons extra-virgin olive oil
- 1 15-ounce can small white beans
- Freshly ground pepper

Directions:

1. Mix tuna, beans, scallions, tomatoes, juice, oil, lemon, pepper, and salt in a medium bowl. Stir gently. Refrigerate until ready to serve.

Nutrition:

- Calories 199
- Fat 8.8 g
- Sodium 555 mg
- Carbohydrates 19.8 g
- Protein 16.5 g

80. Tuna Salad-Stuffed Tomatoes with Arugula

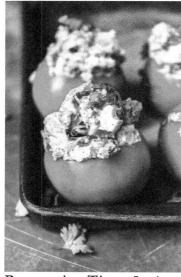

Preparation Time: 5 minutes
Cooking Time: 15 minutes
Servings: 4
Ingredients:

- 1 teaspoon dried thyme

- 3 tablespoons sherry vinegar
- 3 tablespoons extra-virgin olive oil
- 1/3 cup chopped celery
- ¼ teaspoon freshly ground pepper
- 4 large tomatoes
- 8 cups baby arugula
- ¼ cup finely chopped red onion
- ¼ teaspoon salt
- ¼ cup chopped Kalamata olives
- 2 5-oz cans chunk light tuna in olive oil, drained
- 1 can great northern beans, rinsed

Directions:

1. Whisk oil, salt, vinegar, and pepper in an average-sized bowl. Put 3 tablespoons of the dressing in a big bowl and set aside.
2. Slice enough off the top of each tomato to remove the core, chop enough of the tops to equal ½ cup and add to the average-sized bowl. Scoop out the soft tomato tissue using a teaspoon or melon baller and discard the pulp
3. Add tuna, onion, thyme, olives, and celery to the average-sized bowl; gently toss to mix. Fill the scooped tomatoes with the tuna mixture. Add beans and arugula to the gauze in the large bowl and toss to combine. Divide the salad into four plates and top each with a stuffed tomato.

Nutrition:

- Calories 353
- Fat 17.6 g
- Sodium 501 mg
- Carbohydrates 29.9 g
- Protein 19.7 g

81. Curry Vegetable Noodles with Chicken

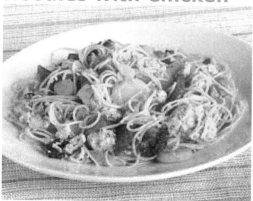

Preparation Time: 15 minutes
Cooking Time: 15 minutes
Servings: 2
Ingredients:

- 600g of zucchini
- 500g chicken fillet
- Pinch of salt and pepper
- 2 tbsp oil
- 150 g of red and yellow cherry tomatoes
- 1 teaspoon curry powder
- 150g fat-free cheese
- 200 ml vegetable broth
- 4 stalk (s) of fresh basil

Directions:
1.   Wash the zucchini, clean, and cut into long thin strips with a spiral cutter. Wash meat, pat dry, and season with salt. Heat 1 tbsp oil in a pan. Roast chicken in it for about 10 minutes until golden brown.
2.   Wash cherry tomatoes and cut them in half. Approximately 3 minutes before the end of the cooking time to the chicken in the pan. Heat 1 tbsp oil in another pan. Sweat curry powder into it, then stir in cream cheese and broth. Flavor the sauce with salt plus pepper and simmer for about 4 minutes.

3.   Wash the basil, shake it dry and pluck the leaves from the stems. Cut small leaves of 3 stems. Remove meat from the pan and cut it into strips. Add tomatoes, basil, and zucchini to the sauce and heat for 2-3 minutes. Serve vegetable noodles and meat on plates and garnish with basil.
Nutrition:
- Calories 376
- Fat 17.2g
- Protein 44.9g
- Sodium 352mg
- Carbohydrate 9.5
- Cholesterol 53mg

82. Eggplant Parmesan Stacks

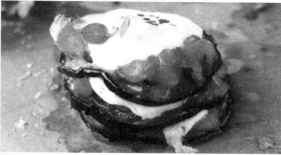

Preparation Time: 15 minutes
Cooking Time: 20 minutes
Servings: 4
Ingredients:

- 1 large eggplant, cut into thick slices
- 2 tablespoons olive oil, divided
- ¼ teaspoon kosher or sea salt
- ¼ teaspoon ground black pepper
- 1 cup panko bread crumbs
- ¼ cup freshly grated Parmesan cheese
- 5 to 6 garlic cloves, minced
- ½ pound fresh mozzarella, sliced
- 1½ cups lower-sodium marinara
- ½ cup fresh basil leaves, torn

Directions:

1. Preheat the oven to 425°F. Coat the eggplant slices in 1 tablespoon olive oil and sprinkle with salt and black pepper. Put on a large baking sheet, then roast for 10 to 12 minutes, until soft with crispy edges. Remove the eggplant and set the oven to low broil.

2. In a bowl, stir the remaining tablespoon of olive oil, bread crumbs, Parmesan cheese, and garlic. Remove the cooled eggplant from the baking sheet and clean it.

3. Create layers on the same baking sheet by stacking a roasted eggplant slice with a slice of mozzarella, a tablespoon of marinara, and a tablespoon of the bread crumb mixture, repeating with 2 layers of each ingredient. Cook under the broiler for 3 to 4 minutes until the cheese is melted and bubbly.

Nutrition:
- Calories: 377
- Fat: 22g
- Sodium: 509mg
- Carbohydrate: 29g
- Protein: 16g

83. Roasted Vegetable Enchiladas

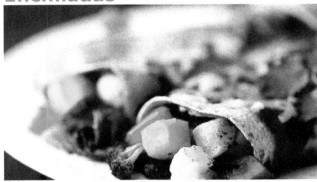

Preparation Time: 15 minutes
Cooking Time: 45 minutes
Servings: 8
Ingredients:
- 2 zucchinis, diced
- 1 red bell pepper, seeded and sliced
- 1 red onion, peeled and sliced
- 2 ears corn
- 2 tablespoons canola oil
- 1 can no-salt-added black beans, drained
- 1½ tablespoons chili powder
- 2 teaspoon ground cumin
- 1/8 teaspoon kosher or sea salt
- ½ teaspoon ground black pepper
- 8 (8-inch) whole-wheat tortillas
- 1 cup Enchilada Sauce or store-bought enchilada sauce
- ½ cup shredded Mexican-style cheese
- ½ cup plain nonfat Greek yogurt
- ½ cup cilantro leaves, chopped

Directions:
1. Preheat oven to 400°F. Place the zucchini, red bell pepper, and red onion on a baking sheet. Place the ears of corn separately on the same baking sheet. Drizzle all with the canola oil and toss to coat. Roast for 10 to 12 minutes until the vegetables are tender. Remove and reduce the temperature to 375°F.

2. Cut the corn from the cob. Transfer the corn kernels, zucchini, red bell pepper, and onion to a bowl and stir in the black beans, chili powder, cumin, salt, and black pepper until combined.

3. Oiled a 9-by-13-inch baking dish with cooking spray. Line up the tortillas in the greased baking dish. Evenly distribute the vegetable bean filling into each tortilla. Pour half of the enchilada sauce and sprinkle half of the shredded cheese on top of the filling.

4. Roll each tortilla into an enchilada shape and place them seam-side down. Pour the remaining enchilada sauce and sprinkle the remaining cheese over the enchiladas. Bake for 25 minutes until the cheese is melted and bubbly. Serve the enchiladas with Greek yogurt and chopped cilantro.

Nutrition:
- Calories: 335
- Fat: 15g
- Sodium: 557mg
- Carbohydrate: 42g
- Protein: 13g

84. Lentil Avocado Tacos

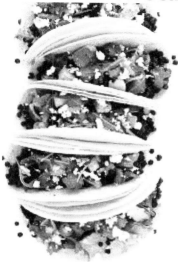

Preparation Time: 15 minutes
Cooking Time: 35 minutes
Servings: 6
Ingredients:

- 1 tablespoon canola oil
- ½ yellow onion, peeled and diced
- 2-3 garlic cloves, minced
- 1½ cups dried lentils
- ½ teaspoon kosher or sea salt
- 3 to 3½ cups unsalted vegetable or chicken stock
- 2½ tablespoons Taco Seasoning or store-bought low-sodium taco seasoning
- 16 (6-inch) corn tortillas, toasted
- 2 ripe avocados, peeled and sliced

Directions:

1. Heat the canola oil in a large skillet or Dutch oven over medium heat. Cook the onion for 4 to 5 minutes, until soft. Mix in the garlic and cook for 30 seconds until fragrant. Then add the lentils, salt, and stock. Bring to a simmer for 25 to 35 minutes, adding additional stock if needed.

2. When there's only a small amount of liquid left in the pan, and the lentils are al dente,

stir in the taco seasoning and let simmer for 1 to 2 minutes. Taste and adjust the seasoning, if necessary. Spoon the lentil mixture into tortillas and serve with the avocado slices.

Nutrition:

- Calories: 400
- Fat: 14g
- Sodium: 336mg
- Carbohydrate: 64g
- Fiber: 15g
- Protein: 16g

85. Tomato & Olive Orecchiette with Basil Pesto

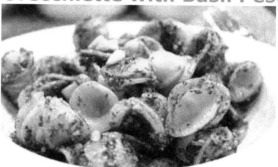

Preparation Time: 15 minutes
Cooking Time: 25 minutes
Servings: 6
Ingredients:

- 12 ounces orecchiette pasta
- 2 tablespoons olive oil
- 1-pint cherry tomatoes, quartered
- ½ cup Basil Pesto or store-bought pesto
- ¼ cup kalamata olives, sliced
- 1 tablespoon dried oregano leaves
- ¼ teaspoon kosher or sea salt
- ½ teaspoon freshly cracked black pepper
- ¼ teaspoon crushed red pepper flakes
- 2 tablespoons freshly grated Parmesan cheese

Directions:

1. Boil a large pot of water. Cook the orecchiette, drain and transfer the pasta to a large nonstick skillet.

2. Put the skillet over medium-low heat, then heat the olive oil. Stir in the cherry tomatoes, pesto, olives, oregano, salt, black pepper, and crushed red pepper flakes. Cook for 8 to 10 minutes, until heated throughout. Serve the pasta with freshly grated Parmesan cheese.

Nutrition:

- Calories: 332
- Fat: 13g
- Sodium: 389mg
- Carbohydrate: 44g
- Protein: 9g

86. Ginger Snaps

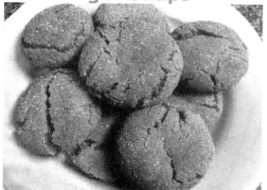

Nutrition:
- Calories: 81
- Fat: 2 g
- Protein: 1 g
- Sodium: 6 mg
- Fiber: 0 g
- Carbohydrates: 14 g
- Sugar: 8 g

Preparation Time: 15 minutes
Cooking Time: 10 minutes
Servings: 18
Ingredients:
- 4 tablespoons unsalted butter
- 1/2 cup light brown sugar
- 2 tablespoons molasses
- 1 egg white
- 21/2 teaspoons ground ginger
- 1/4 teaspoon ground allspice
- 1 teaspoon sodium-free baking soda
- 1/2 cup unbleached all-purpose flour
- 12 cup white whole-wheat flour
- 1 tablespoon sugar

Directions:
1. Heat the oven to 375°F. Put aside a baking sheet with parchment paper. Put the butter, sugar, plus molasses into a mixing bowl and beat well.
2. Mix the egg white, ginger, and allspice. Mix in the baking soda, then put the flours, then beat.
3. Roll the dough into small balls. Put the balls on a prepared baking sheet and press down using a glass dipped in the tablespoon sugar.
4. Once the glass presses on the dough, it will moisten sufficiently to coat with sugar. Bake for 10 minutes. Let it cool, then serve.

87. Carrot Cake Cookies

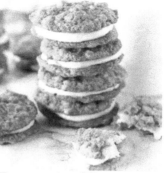

Preparation Time: 15 minutes
Cooking Time: 12 minutes
Servings: 36
Ingredients:
- 3 medium carrots, shredded
- 11/2 cups white whole-wheat flour
- 3/4 cup oat flour
- 3/4 cup light brown sugar
- 1 egg white
- 1/3 cup canola oil
- 1 tablespoon pure vanilla extract
- 1 teaspoon sodium-free baking powder
- 11/2 teaspoons ground cinnamon
- 1/2 teaspoon ground nutmeg
- 1/4 teaspoon ground ginger
- 1/8 teaspoon ground cloves

Directions:
1. Preheat oven to 375°F. Prepare and line a baking sheet with parchment paper and set

aside. Place all the ingredients into a mixing bowl and stir well to combine. The dough will be quite sticky.

2. Put onto a lined baking sheet. Bake for 12 minutes. Remove, then transfer cookies to a wire rack to cool. Store in an airtight container.

Nutrition:

- Calories: 67
- Fat: 2 g
- Protein: 1 g
- Sodium: 7 mg
- Fiber: 0 g
- Carbohydrates: 10 g
- Sugar: 4 g

88. Grilled Pineapple Strips

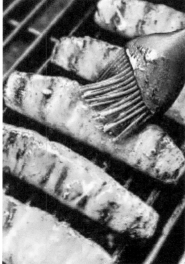

Preparation Time: 15 minutes
Cooking Time: 5 minutes
Servings: 6
Ingredients:

- Vegetable oil
- Dash of iodized salt
- 1 pineapple
- 1 tablespoon lime juice extract
- 1 tablespoon olive oil
- 1 tablespoon raw honey
- 3 tablespoons brown sugar

Directions:

1. Peel the pineapple, remove the eyes of the fruit, and discard the core. Slice lengthwise, forming six wedges. Mix the rest of the ingredients in a bowl until blended.

2. Brush the coating mixture on the pineapple (reserve some for basting). Grease an oven or outdoor grill rack with vegetable oil.

3. Place the pineapple wedges on the grill rack and heat for a few minutes per side until golden brownish, basting it frequently with a reserved glaze. Serve on a platter.

Nutrition:

- Calories 97
- Fats 2 g
- Carbohydrates 20 g
- Sodium 2 mg
- Sugar 17 g
- Fibers 1 g
- Proteins 1 g

89. Raspberry Peach Pancake

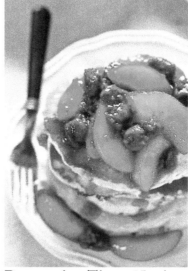

Preparation Time: 15 minutes
Cooking Time: 30 minutes

Servings: 4
Ingredients:

- ½ teaspoon sugar
- ½ cup raspberries
- ½ cup fat-free milk
- ½ cup all-purpose flour
- ¼ cup vanilla yogurt
- 1/8 teaspoon iodized salt
- 1 tablespoon butter
- 2 medium peeled, thinly sliced peaches
- 3 lightly beaten organic eggs

Directions:

1.   Preheat oven to 400 °F. Toss peaches and raspberries with sugar in a bowl. Melt butter on a 9-inch round baking plate. Mix eggs, milk, plus salt in a small bowl until blended; whisk in the flour.

2.   Remove the round baking plate from the oven, tilt to coat the bottom and sides with the melted butter; pour in the flour mixture.

3.   Put it in the oven until it becomes brownish and puffed. Remove the pancake from the oven. Serve immediately with more raspberries and vanilla yogurt.

Nutrition:

- Calories 199
- Sodium 173 mg
- Fats 7 g
- Cholesterol 149 g
- Carbohydrates 25 g
- Sugar 11 g
- Fibers 3 g
- Proteins 9 g

90. Apple Dumplings

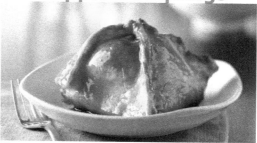

Preparation Time: 10 minutes
Cooking Time: 30 minutes
Servings: 6
Ingredients:
Dough:

- 1 tablespoon butter
- 1 teaspoon honey
- 1 cup whole-wheat flour
- 2 tablespoons buckwheat flour
- 2 tablespoons rolled oats
- 2 tablespoons brandy or apple liquor

Apple filling:

- 6 large tart apples, thinly sliced
- 1 teaspoon nutmeg
- 2 tablespoons honey
- Zest of one lemon

Directions:

1.   Warm oven to heat at 350 degrees F. Combine flours with oats, honey, and butter in a food processor. Pulse this mixture a few times, then stir in apple liquor or brandy. Mix until it forms a ball. Wrap it in a plastic sheet.

2.   Refrigerate for 2 hours. Mix apples with honey, nutmeg, and lemon zest, then set it aside. Spread the dough into ¼ inch thick sheet. Cut it into 8-inch circles and layer the greased muffin cups with the dough circles.

3.   Divide the apple mixture into the muffin cups and seal the dough from the top. Bake for 30 minutes at 350 degrees F until golden brown. Enjoy.

Nutrition:

- Calories 178
- Fat 5.7 g
- Cholesterol 15 mg
- Sodium 114 mg
- Carbs 12.4 g
- Fiber 0.2g
- Sugar 15 g
- Protein 9.1 g

91. Berries Marinated in Balsamic Vinegar

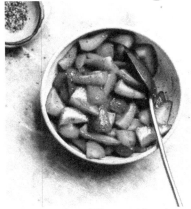

Preparation Time: 10 minutes
Cooking Time: 0 minutes
Servings: 2
Ingredients:

- 1/4 cup balsamic vinegar
- 2 tablespoons brown sugar
- 1 teaspoon vanilla extract
- 1/2 cup sliced strawberries
- 1/2 cup blueberries
- 1/2 cup raspberries
- 2 shortbread biscuits

Directions:
1. Combine balsamic vinegar, vanilla, and brown sugar in a small bowl. Toss strawberries with raspberries and blueberries in a bowl. Pour the vinegar mixture on top and marinate them for 15 minutes. Serve immediately.
Nutrition:

- Calories 176
- Fat 11.9 g
- Cholesterol 78 mg
- Sodium 79 mg
- Carbs 33 g
- Fiber 1.1 g
- Sugar 10.3 g
- Protein 13 g

92. Lemon Pudding Cakes

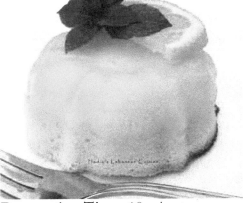

Preparation Time: 10 minutes
Cooking Time: 40 minutes
Servings: 4
Ingredients:

- 2 eggs
- 1/4 teaspoon salt
- 3/4 cup sugar
- 1 cup skim milk
- 1/3 cup freshly squeezed lemon juice
- 3 tablespoons all-purpose flour
- 1 tablespoon finely grated lemon peel
- 1 tablespoon melted butter

Directions:
1. Warm oven at 350 degrees F. Grease the custard cups with cooking oil. Whisk egg whites with salt and ¼ cup sugar in a mixer until it forms stiff peaks. Beat egg yolks with ½ cup sugar until mixed.
2. Stir in lemon juice, milk, butter, flour, and lemon peel. Mix it until smooth. Fold in the

egg white mixture. Divide the batter into the custard cups. Bake them for 40 minutes until golden from the top. Serve.

Nutrition:

- Calories 174
- Fat 10.2 g
- Cholesterol 120 mg
- Sodium 176 mg
- Carbs 19 g
- Fiber 1.9 g
- Sugar 11.4 g
- Protein 12.8 g

93. Mixed Berry Whole-Grain Coffee Cake

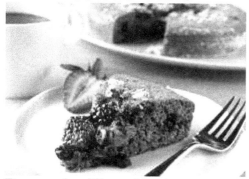

Preparation Time: 10 minutes
Cooking Time: 30 minutes
Servings: 6
Ingredients:

- 1/2 cup of skim milk
- 1 tbsp vinegar
- 2 tbsp canola oil
- 1 tsp vanilla
- 1 egg
- 1/3 cup of packed brown sugar
- 1 cup of whole-wheat pastry flour
- 1/2 tsp baking soda
- 1/2 tsp ground cinnamon
- 1/8 tsp salt
- 1 cup of frozen mixed berries
- 1/4 cup of low-fat granola, slightly crushed

Directions:

1. Warm oven to heat at 350 degrees F. Grease an 8-inch baking pan with cooking spray and dust it with flour. Combine milk with vanilla, oil, vinegar, brown sugar, and egg until smooth.
2. Add baking soda, cinnamon, salt, and flour. Mix well. Fold in half of the berries and transfer the batter to the pan. Top it with the berries and granola. Bake for 30 minutes until golden brown. Serve.

Nutrition:

- Calories 135
- Fat 24g
- Cholesterol 61 mg
- Sodium 562 mg
- Carbs 23 g
- Fiber 1.7 g
- Sugar 39 g
- Protein 11g

94. Strawberries and Cream Cheese Crepes

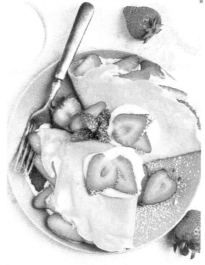

Preparation Time: 10 minutes
Cooking Time: 10 minutes
Servings: 2
Ingredients:

- 4 tbsp cream cheese, softened
- 2 tbsp powdered sugar, sifted
- 2 tsp vanilla extract
- 2 pre-packaged crepes, each about 8 inches in diameter
- 8 strawberries, hulled and sliced

Directions:

1. Set the oven to heat at 325 degrees F. Grease a baking dish with cooking spray. Mix cream cheese with vanilla plus powdered sugar in a mixer. Spread the cream cheese mixture on each crepe and top it with 2 tablespoons of strawberries.

2. Roll the crepes and place them in the baking dish. Bake them for 10 minutes until golden brown. Garnish as desired. Serve.

Nutrition:

- Calories 144
- Fat 4.9 g
- Cholesterol 11 mg
- Sodium 13 mg
- Carbs 19.3 g
- Fiber 1.9 g
- Sugar 9.7 g
- Protein 3.4 g

95. Chocolate Cake in A Mug

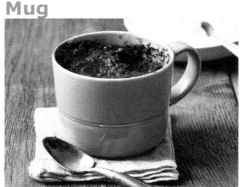

Preparation Time: 5 minutes
Cooking Time: 1 minute
Servings: 1
Ingredients:

- 3 tablespoons white whole-wheat flour
- 2 tablespoons unsweetened cocoa powder
- 2 teaspoons sugar
- 1/8 teaspoon baking powder
- 1 egg white
- ½ teaspoon olive oil
- 3 tablespoons nonfat or low-fat milk
- ½ teaspoon vanilla extract
- Cooking spray

Directions:

1. Place the flour, cocoa, sugar, and baking powder in a small bowl and whisk until combined. Then add in the egg white, olive oil, milk, and vanilla extract, and mix to combine.

2. Oiled a mug with cooking spray and pour batter into the mug. Microwave on high for 60 seconds or until set. Serve.

Nutrition:

- Calories: 217
- Fat: 4 g
- Cholesterol: 1 mg
- Sodium: 139 mg
- Carbs: 35 g

- Fiber: 7 g
- Sugar: 12 g
- Protein: 11 g

96. Peanut Butter Banana "Ice Cream"

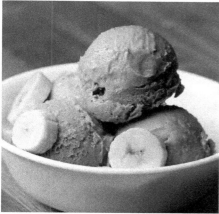

Preparation Time: 10 minutes
Cooking Time: 0 minutes
Servings: 4
Ingredients:

- 2 tablespoons peanut butter
- 4 bananas, very ripe, peeled, and sliced into ½-inch rings

Directions:

1. On a large baking sheet or plate, spread the banana slices in an even layer. Freeze for 1 to 2 hours. Puree the frozen banana until it forms a smooth and creamy mixture in a food processor or blender, scraping down the bowl as needed.
2. Add the peanut butter, pureeing until just combined. For a soft-serve ice cream consistency, serve immediately. For a harder consistency, place the ice cream in the freezer for a few hours before serving.

Nutrition:

- Calories: 153
- Fat: 4 g
- Sodium: 4 mg
- Carbs: 29 g
- Fiber: 4 g
- Sugar: 15 g
- Protein: 3 g

97. Banana-Cashew Cream Mousse

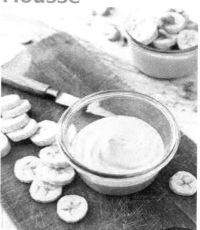

Preparation Time: 55 minutes
Cooking Time: 0 minutes
Servings: 2
Ingredients:

- ½ cup cashews, presoaked
- 1 tablespoon honey
- 1 teaspoon vanilla extract
- 1 cup plain nonfat Greek yogurt
- 1 large banana, sliced (reserve 4 slices for garnish)

Directions:

1. Put the cashews in your small bowl, then cover with 1 cup of water. Dip at room temperature for 2 to 3 hours. Drain, rinse and set aside. Place honey, vanilla extract, cashews, and bananas in a blender or food processor.
2. Blend until smooth. Place mixture in a medium bowl. Fold in yogurt, mix well. Cover, then chill for 45 minutes. Portion mousse into 2 serving bowls. Garnish each with 2 banana slices.

Nutrition:

- Calories: 329
- Fat: 14 g
- Sodium: 64 mg
- Carbs: 37 g
- Fiber: 3 g
- Sugar: 24 g
- Protein: 17 g

98. Grilled Plums with Vanilla Bean Frozen Yogurt

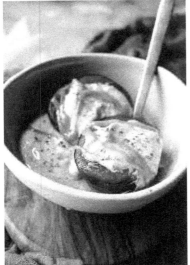

Preparation Time: 10 minutes
Cooking Time: 15 minutes
Servings: 4
Ingredients:
- 4 large plums, sliced in half and pitted
- 1 tablespoon olive oil
- 1 tablespoon honey
- 1 teaspoon ground cinnamon
- 2 cups vanilla bean frozen yogurt

Directions:
1. Preheat the grill to medium heat. Brush the plum halves with olive oil. Grill, flesh-side down, for 4 to 5 minutes, then flip and cook for another 4 to 5 minutes, until just tender.
2. Mix the honey plus cinnamon in a small bowl. Scoop the frozen yogurt into 4 bowls. Place 2 plum halves in each bowl and drizzle each with the cinnamon-honey mixture.

Nutrition:
- Calories: 192
- Fat: 8 g
- Sodium: 63 mg
- Carbs: 30 g
- Fiber: 1 g
- Sugar: 28 g
- Protein: 3 g

99. Key Lime Cherry "Nice" Cream

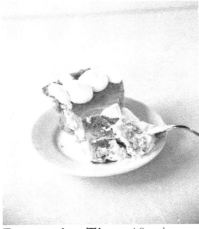

Preparation Time: 10 minutes
Cooking Time: 15 minutes
Servings: 4
Ingredients:
- 4 frozen bananas, peeled
- 1 cup frozen dark sweet cherries
- Zest and juice of 1 lime, divided
- ½ teaspoon vanilla extract
- ¼ teaspoon kosher or sea salt

Directions:
1. Blend the ingredients in a food processor and enjoy a frozen treat. Place the bananas, cherries, lime juice, vanilla extract, and salt in a food processor and purée until smooth, scraping the sides as needed.
2. Transfer the "nice" cream to bowls and top with the lime zest. For leftovers, place the "nice" cream in airtight containers and store them in the freezer for up to 1 month. Let thaw for 30 minutes until it reaches a soft-serve ice cream texture.

Nutrition:

- Calories: 150
- Fat: 0 g
- Sodium: 147 mg
- Carbs: 37 g
- Fiber: 4 g
- Sugar: 21 g
- Protein: 2 g

100. Oatmeal Dark Chocolate Chip Peanut Butter Cookies

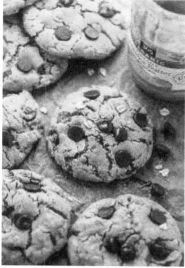

Preparation Time: 15 minutes
Cooking Time: 10 minutes
Servings: 24
Ingredients:

- 1½ cups natural creamy peanut butter
- ½ cup dark brown sugar
- 2 large eggs
- 1 cup old-fashioned rolled oats
- 1 teaspoon baking soda
- ½ teaspoon kosher or sea salt
- ½ cup dark chocolate chips

Directions:

1. Preheat the oven to 350°F. Line a baking sheet with parchment paper. Whip the peanut butter in the bowl of a stand mixer until very smooth. Continue beating and add the brown sugar, then one egg at a time, until fluffy.

2. Beat in the oats, baking soda, and salt until combined. Fold in the dark chocolate chips. Put the cookie dough on the baking sheet, about 2 inches apart. Bake for 8 to 10 minutes, depending on your preferred level of doneness.

Nutrition:

- Calories: 152
- Fat: 10 g
- Sodium: 131 mg
- Carbs: 12 g
- Fiber: 2 g
- Sugar: 8 g
- Protein: 4 g

101. Healthy Blueberry & Banana Muffins

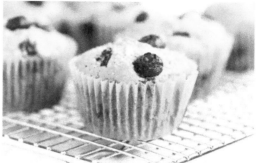

Preparation Time: 30 minutes
Cooking Time: 25 minutes
Servings: 12
Ingredients:

- 3/4 cup mashed ripe banana
- 3/4 cup + 2 tbsp almond milk, unsweetened
- 1 teaspoon apple cider vinegar
- 1/4 cup pure maple syrup
- 1 teaspoon pure vanilla extract
- 1/4 cup coconut oil, melted
- 1/2 teaspoon baking soda
- 2 teaspoons baking powder

- 4 tablespoons coconut sugar
- 1 1/2 teaspoons cinnamon
- 2 cups white spelt flour
- 1 1/4 cups of blueberries
- 1/2 cup walnut halves, chopped

Directions:

1.   Prepare lined 12-muffin tin with muffin liners and preheat oven to 350oF. In a large mixing bowl, whisk well-mashed bananas, almond milk, vinegar, maple syrup, vanilla, melted coconut oil, baking soda, baking powder, coconut sugar, and cinnamon.

2.   Whisk well until thoroughly incorporated. Fold in spelt flour. Add blueberries and walnut halves. Evenly divide batter into prepared muffin tins. Bake for 25 minutes. Cool completely. Serve.

Nutrition:

- Calories: 226.5
- Protein: 5g
- Carbs: 33.4g
- Fat: 8.1g
- Sodium: 67mg

102. Mango Rice Pudding

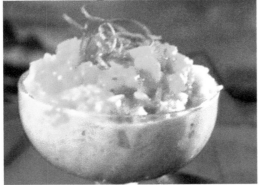

Preparation Time: 15 minutes
Cooking Time: 35 minutes
Servings: 4
Ingredients:

- ½ teaspoon ground cinnamon
- ¼ teaspoon iodized salt
- 1 teaspoon vanilla extract
- 1 cup long-grain uncooked brown rice
- 2 mediums ripe, peeled, cored mango
- 1 cup vanilla soymilk
- 2 tablespoons sugar
- 2 cups of water

Directions:

1.   Bring saltwater to a boil in a saucepan to cook rice; after a few minutes, simmer covered for 30-35 minutes until the rice absorbs the water. Mash the mango with a mortar and pestle or stainless-steel fork.

2.   Pour milk, sugar, cinnamon, and the mashed mango into the rice; cook uncovered on low heat, stirring frequently. Remove the mango rice pudding from the heat, then stir in the vanilla soymilk. Serve immediately.

Nutrition:

- Calories 275
- Sodium 176 mg
- Fats 3 g
- Carbohydrates 58 mg
- Sugar 20 g
- Fibers 3 g

103. Choco Banana Cake

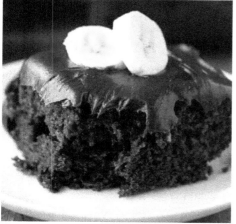

Preparation Time: 15 minutes
Cooking Time: 30 minutes
Servings: 18
Ingredients:

- ½ cup semisweet dark chocolate
- ½ cup brown sugar
- ½ teaspoon baking soda
- ¼ cup unsweetened cocoa powder
- ¼ cup canola oil
- ¾ cup soymilk
- 1 large egg
- 1 egg white
- 1 large, ripe, mashed banana
- 1 tablespoon lemon juice extract
- 1 teaspoon vanilla extract
- 2 cups all-purpose flour

Directions:

1. Preheat the oven to 350 °F. Coat a baking pan with a non-stick spray. Whisk brown sugar, flour, baking soda, and cocoa powder in a bowl.
2. In another bowl, whisk bananas, lemon juice extract, vanilla extract, oil, soymilk, egg, and egg whites. Create a hole in the flour mixture's core or center, then pour in the banana mixture and mix in the dark chocolate.

3. Stir all the ingredients with a spoon until thoroughly blended; spoon the batter onto the baking pan. Place in the oven and bake for 25-30 minutes until the center springs back when pressed lightly using your fingertips.

Nutrition:

- Calories 150
- Sodium 52 mg
- Cholesterol 12 mg
- Fats 3 g
- Carbohydrates 27 g
- Proteins 3 g

104. Chewy Pumpkin Oatmeal Raisin Cookies

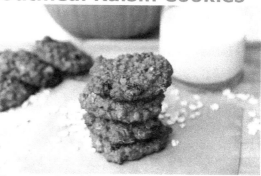

Preparation Time: 15 minutes
Cooking Time: 16 minutes
Servings: 48
Ingredients:

- 1 cup pumpkin purée
- 12/3 cups sugar
- 2 tablespoons molasses
- 11/2 teaspoons pure vanilla extract
- 2/3 cup canola oil
- 1 tablespoon ground flaxseed
- 2 teaspoons Ener-G Baking Soda Substitute
- 1 teaspoon ground cinnamon
- 1/2 teaspoon ground nutmeg
- 1 cup unbleached all-purpose flour
- 1 cup white whole-wheat flour

- 11/3 cups rolled or quick oats
- 1 cup seedless raisins

Directions:

1. Preheat oven to 350°F. Spray 2 baking sheets lightly with oil and set aside. Measure the ingredients into a large mixing bowl and stir using a rubber spatula.

2. Scoop batter out by tablespoons—a small retractable ice cream scoop works wonderfully here—and place on the prepared baking sheets.

3. Put sheets on the middle rack in the oven and bake for 16 minutes. Remove, then transfer cookies to a wire rack to cool. Repeat the process with the remaining batter. Cool and serve.

Nutrition:

- Calories: 97
- Fat: 3 g
- Protein: 1 g
- Sodium: 1 mg
- Fiber: 0.6 g
- Carbohydrates: 16 g
- Sugar: 9 g

105. Easy Apple Crisp

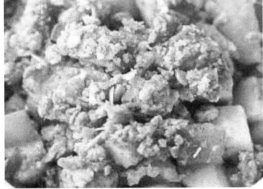

Preparation Time: 15 minutes
Cooking Time: 25 minutes
Servings: 8
Ingredients:

- 6 medium apples
- 1 tablespoon lemon juice
- 1/3 cup sugar
- 1/2 cup rolled or quick oats
- 1/2 cup white whole-wheat flour
- 1/2 cup light brown sugar
- 1 tablespoon pure vanilla extract
- 1 teaspoon ground cinnamon
- 1/2 teaspoon ground ginger
- 3 tablespoons unsalted butter

Directions:

1. Preheat oven to 425°F. Take out a 2-quart baking pan and set it aside. Slice each apple into 16 wedges. Put into a mixing bowl, place the lemon juice and sugar, and toss well to coat.

2. Turn the batter out into the baking pan, then set aside. Place the oats, flour, sugar, vanilla, and spices into a mixing bowl and stir to combine.

3. Slice the butter into the mixture using your hands and process until a wet crumb has formed. Sprinkle mixture over the fruit. Bake for 25 minutes. Remove, then let it cool and serve.

Nutrition:

- Calories: 232
- Fat: 5 g
- Protein: 2 g
- Sodium: 5 mg
- Fiber: 2 g
- Carbohydrates: 46 g
- Sugar: 34 g

106. Mango Crumble

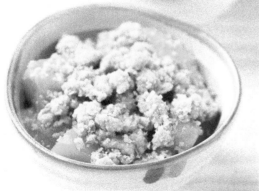

Preparation Time: 15 minutes
Cooking Time: 25 minutes
Servings: 8
Ingredients:

- 2 barely ripe mangoes
- 2 tablespoons light brown sugar
- 1 tablespoon cornstarch
- 11/2 teaspoons minced fresh ginger
- 1/2 cup unbleached all-purpose flour
- 1/2 cup white whole-wheat flour
- 1/2 cup sugar
- 1 teaspoon ground cinnamon
- 1/4 teaspoon ground ginger
- 3 tablespoons unsalted butter

Directions:

1. Preheat oven to 375°F. Take out an 8-inch square baking pan and set it aside. Peel mangoes and cut into 1-inch chunks. Place in a mixing bowl.

2. Add the brown sugar, cornstarch, and minced ginger and toss to coat. Put the batter out into the baking pan and spread to even. In another bowl, whisk the flours, sugar, cinnamon, and ginger.

3. Slice the butter into pieces, and put it in the bowl. Work the butter into the mixture using your hands until it resembles damp sand and sticks when squeezed. Sprinkle mixture evenly over the fruit.

4. Bake for 25 minutes, until fruit is tender. Remove and put on a wire rack to cool. Serve warm or cool.

Nutrition:

- Calories: 190
- Fat: 5 g
- Protein: 3 g
- Sodium: 3 mg
- Fiber: 2 g
- Carbohydrates: 37 g
- Sugar: 23 g

107. Homemade Banana Ice Cream

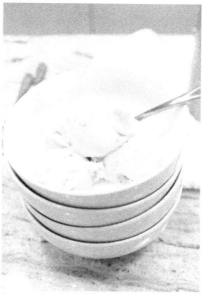

Preparation Time: 5 minutes
Cooking Time: 0 minutes
Servings: 4
Ingredients:

- 4 ripe bananas

Directions:

1. Place bananas in the freezer and freeze until solid. Remove bananas from the freezer, peel, and slice into chunks. Pulse chunks into a blender or food processor. Scoop mixture out and serve immediately.

Nutrition:

- Calories: 105
- Fat: 0 g
- Protein: 1 g
- Sodium: 1 mg
- Fiber: 3 g
- Carbohydrates: 26 g
- Sugar: 14 g

Conclusion

Thank you for making it through to the end of this book. Let's hope it was useful, informative, and able to provide you with all of the tools you need to achieve your goals, whatever they may be.

The next step is to begin your DASH diet with a healthy lifestyle. Your average American diet mostly comprises food options that are not healthy. As a result, you may be facing the threat of lifestyle diseases. If you're worried about your health, consider following the DASH diet. The DASH diet is your gateway to optimum health and lifestyle.

This diet has been endorsed by the National Institutes of Health along with backing from various health organizations, among them the American Heart Association and Mayo Clinic. Its success is based on realistic nutritional advice that includes the following:

- Increasing your consumption of fiber lets you maintain steady blood pressure while also losing weight.

- Reducing your intake of sodium goes a long way in minimizing the risk of hypertension.

- Minimizing saturated fat as well as trans-fat will increase your heart health, raise your HDL cholesterol, lower your LDL cholesterol and minimize the risks of heart disease.

- Increasing your intake of healthy fats by eating seeds, fish, nuts, avocado, and other foods rich in Omega 3.

Thank you for getting here. I wish you a good journey!

CPSIA information can be obtained
at www.ICGtesting.com
Printed in the USA
LVHW061106260521
688558LV00002B/9